Praise for Inna Segal's

THE SECRET OF
LIFE WELLNESS

"The great sages have been telling us what Inna Segal shares in her new book,
The Secret of Life Wellness. What is on your mind, [and] in your heart and soul matters, and
relates to your health and life experience. Inna shares universal truths we can all
learn from, as she presents them in a way that is practical, inspiring and powerful.
Our lives, past and present, are stored within us, and must be confronted and healed."
Bernie Siegel, MD, author of *A Book of Miracles* and *Faith, Hope & Healing*

"*The Secret of Life Wellness* offers fresh insights and powerful techniques that will impact every
area of your life. Inna Segal is a true visionary who shares important wisdom for our times.
If you want to create a life filled with happiness, love, and prosperity,
I highly recommend this book."
Marci Shimoff, author of *Happy for No Reason* and *Love for No Reason*

"Inna Segal has written a clarified and inclusive guide to wellness. *The Secret of Life Wellness*
is a wonderful invitation to wholeness. Highly recommended!"
Jeff Brown, author of *Soulshaping: A Journey of Self-Creation*

"Inna Segal is a powerful visionary and healer whose work is only surpassed by the heart she
brings to it. *The Secret of Life Wellness* outlines the divine elixir for bringing one's experience
into a state of grace-filled well-being. This book is a 'must have' for your journey."
Simran Singh, publisher of *11:11 Magazine*, author of *Conversations with the Universe*

"To truly understand the secrets to Life's Big Questions, read Inna's book,
The Secret of Life Wellness. It's sensational!"
Thom Hartmann, author of *Rebooting the American Dream*

"If you want to find easy, effective intuitive methods that apply to a wide range of life's tasks
and undertakings, this is the book for you! In *The Secret of Life Wellness*, Inna Segal gives
many tips and techniques that can strengthen your intuition and turn your life into a spiritual
practice. She shows you how powerful your imagination can be!"
Penney Peirce, author of *Leap of Perception, Frequency* and *The Intuitive Way*

THE
SECRET
OF
LIFE
WELLNESS

THE ESSENTIAL GUIDE TO LIFE'S BIG QUESTIONS

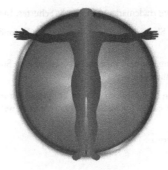

INNA SEGAL

FOREWORD BY MICHAEL BERNARD BECKWITH

ATRIA PAPERBACK
New York London Toronto Sydney New Delhi

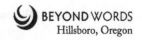
BEYOND WORDS
Hillsboro, Oregon

ATRIA PAPERBACK
A Division of Simon & Schuster, Inc.
1230 Avenue of the Americas
New York, NY 10020

BEYOND WORDS
20827 N.W. Cornell Road, Suite 500
Hillsboro, Oregon 97124-9808
503-531-8700 / 503-531-8773 fax
www.beyondword.com

This publication contains the opinions and ideas of its author. It is intended to provide helpful and informative material on the subjects addressed in the publication. It is sold with the understanding that the author and publisher are not engaged in rendering medical, health, or any other kind of personal professional services in the book. The reader should consult his or her medical, health, or other competent professional before adopting any of the suggestions in this book or drawing inferences from it. The author and publisher specifically disclaim all responsibility for any liability, loss, or risk, personal or otherwise, which is incurred as a consequence, directly or indirectly, of the use and application of any of the contents of this book.

Managing editor: Lindsay S. Brown
Editor: Sheila Ashdown
Copyeditor: Henry Covey
Proofreader: Jennifer Weaver-Neist
Design: Devon Smith
Composition: William H. Brunson Typography Services

First Atria Paperback/Beyond Words trade paperback edition September 2013

For more information about special discounts for bulk purchases, please contact Simon & Schuster Special Sales at 1-866-506-1949 or business@simonandschuster.com.

The Simon & Schuster Speakers Bureau can bring authors to your live event. For more information or to book an event, contact the Simon & Schuster Speakers Bureau at 1-866-248-3049 or visit our website at www.simonspeakers.com.

Manufactured in the United States of America

10 9 8 7 6 5 4

Library of Congress Cataloging-in-Publication Data

Segal, Inna.
  The secret of life wellness : the essential guide to life's big questions / by Inna Segal.
     pages   cm
  1. Intuition.   2. Interpersonal relations.   3. Self-realization.   I. Title.
  BF315.5.S44   2013
  158—dc22
                                                                    2013007794

ISBN 978-1-58270-286-5
ISBN 978-1-4767-2964-0 (ebook)

The corporate mission of Beyond Words Publishing, Inc.: *Inspire to Integrity*

The Secret of Life Wellness rests in the hands of Divinity
and is dedicated to the Infinite Love within us all.

I also dedicate this work to my husband, Paul, who inspires, supports,
and loves me unconditionally.

CONTENTS

Contents

FOREWORD

Intuition—we all innately possess it, yet intuition stands low on the totem of qualities society and education encourage us to consciously cultivate. Most of us choose to rely upon those considered to have the "gift" of intuition. However, this is a fallacy because intuition is not a gift. Each of us has been innately endowed with the power of intuition, although its development varies within each individual.

It would not be an exaggeration to say that on a daily basis we experience unexplained feelings we label as "hunches," when in truth they point to the existence of underdeveloped intuition yearning to find expression in, through, and as us. In *The Secret of Life Wellness*, Inna Segal teaches us how to access our intuition and apply it to all aspects of our lives.

Intuition cannot be explained scientifically because the very phenomenon is unscientific; it is beyond logic. However, the collective conviction within our global society is that answers to the challenges of twenty-first-century living are to be found in the empirical evidence provided by science and technology. Never mind that worldwide societal structures—including governments, armed forces, and allopathic medicine, to name a few—covertly turn to intuitives for their psychic input, while everyday citizens turn to shamans, *curanderas*, and readers of all types (including animal intuitives) for panaceas and answers. Even great scientists reach a point where they must wait for a hunch, that intuitive flash that arises from within. Intuition, one of the most subtle energies within us, is direct perception. What can be more practical and accurate?

The important thing to realize is that intuition goes beyond the rationalizing, analyzing, intellectual mind that is often held hostage by the five senses and perceptual limitations. Logic is how the mind interprets reality; intuition is how the inner spirit experiences reality. Intuition takes you beyond mind into the clarity of crystal-clear knowingness. The wisdom of the physical body is instinct, and the wisdom of soul-consciousness is intuition.

Through her direct experience, Inna wisely encourages us by saying, "The truth is that intuition is natural and available to all who are willing to invest the appropriate time and energy to hone it." Intuition is one of the most down-to-earth and vital qualities to develop—one that assists us in all aspects of our lives. The good news is that it does not have to be imported or transplanted from some outer source. It is already within us, just as the acorn tree lives within the seed, awaiting proper nourishment so that it may blossom.

Intuition is your inner "seeing" eye that always directs you on the right course. It has no methodological procedure; it simply catches the pure truth. You may trustfully clean the lens of your inner intuitive eye by accepting Inna's invitation to participate in your own healing, which means taking responsibility for growing up and becoming spiritually mature—a vital need on the collective level at this juncture in our human history. Through the practice of her teachings, you will nourish and support your natural intuitive gift. Through the strength found in the gentleness of self-love, *The Secret of Life Wellness* will ultimately guide you into the all-knowing power of intuition, heaven's own kiss of inspiration.

—Michael Bernard Beckwith

PREFACE

The Secret of Life Wellness is about healing, transforming, and loving your life! My intention is to inspire you to be a visionary and to apply principles and practices of wellness and evolution to yourself and your life.

A great deal of the information, experiences, and processes contained in this book are based on a new modality that I have created called Visionary Intuitive Healing®, which came about after my own life-altering healing experience. After healing severe back pain, digestive problems, psoriasis, and anxiety, I discovered my ability to not only tune in to my own physical body but to also have access to my soul's wisdom. With practice, I developed a capacity to accurately "see," sense, and receive insights into another person's physical, emotional, and energetic state. I could perceive why people had particular illnesses based on the way they lived their lives and processed information.

My ability to perceive the subtle realms has also enabled me to compile highly effective yet simple processes that can help people heal physical problems, release limiting emotions, work with colors and energy, and access and reprogram their subconscious mind. My interest has always been to help people develop their intuition and practically apply it to their lives, as well as to assist them with their self-healing, transformation, and evolution—to be a visionary.

My Inspiration for the Book

The Secret of Life Wellness is based on my many years of teaching Visionary Intuitive Healing® workshops, seeing clients, working with doctors and other health practitioners, research, personal experience, travel, and receiving higher guidance. I felt inspired to write this book after being asked many recurring questions during my seminars, in healing sessions, via email, and from social and traditional media.

Over the years, I found that it didn't matter in which part of the world I was teaching; people's questions about life's deepest issues were almost identical. The majority were interested in how their thoughts and emotions affected their health, and wondered if they had the power to heal themselves. Releasing stress and worry was a hot subject, as well as following your purpose and becoming successful. People wanted to know how to apply my teachings to the various areas of their life.

I have received thousands of questions, and I have compiled them into various categories. As many of the questions were similar, I cut them down to the twenty-one most-asked-about topics and then wrote a composite question to cover the essential information people wanted to know. Each chapter includes my insights, real-life examples, practical advice, and transformational processes.

Just as my previous book, *The Secret Language of Your Body*, has been an important guide for many to improve their health, my intention for *The Secret of Life Wellness* is for it to be a practical resource for transforming important areas of people's lives. This includes pertinent topics such as loving yourself, improving your relationships, attaining your ideal weight, strengthening your intuition, raising confident children, creating financial abundance, and many others. I always emphasize that the state of your body reflects your experience of life, and your life wellness mirrors your physical wellness. When there is an improvement in one, the other is inevitably and greatly enhanced.

INTRODUCTION

The Secret of Life Wellness is not only a guidebook of accessible solutions for some of life's most prevalent questions, but it is also part of a growing world movement encouraging and teaching people to be visionaries—to tune in to their own wisdom and transform their lives. It is an interactive experience containing powerful processes and healing frequencies that lead people to a greater life experience. More of us than ever before are ready for an epic shift of consciousness, both individually and as a people. We are ready to find new ways of living, which work in practical, loving, peaceful, united, and healthy ways. We are ready to have more soulful, spiritual, conscious solutions to both personal and global challenges. We need a new way!

My aim throughout this book (just as in my other books, audio programs, card decks, videos, and workshops) is to gently and persistently encourage you to trust your intuitive guidance and lead you toward an inspired, courageous, and meaningful life.

Over the years, countless students have asked me where they could learn more about the topics I have written about in the chapters that lie ahead. While at times I could direct them to important works I had read, they often complained that the books were difficult to find or didn't exist in their particular language, or that they simply did not have time to read the quantity of books I suggested. Also many of my discoveries did not exist in other people's books and came from my ability to see into people's bodies and energy fields, as well as through my own experiences, visions, and voice of inner guidance.

Thus, I am thrilled to offer such a delicious diversity of subjects to you, all in one book. These include topics as sensitive and varied as attracting a loving partner, preparing for pregnancy, raising more confident and happier children, and many others. While some subjects may only touch you during certain periods of your life, they are all important, so I urge you to read each chapter, as it may contain significant knowledge and processes for your healing and evolution.

The information in this book is part of a movement that is encouraging us to be softer with ourselves; to listen to our body's intuitive messages; to live a more peaceful, soulful, healthier life; to relax; and to connect to and look after nature.

How to Use This Book

In this book, I discuss the various ways you can connect to your intuition, open your heart, listen to your soul, and create a life of wellness. Although you don't necessarily have to read this book in the order it is written, you may find this helpful, as there are many important threads that link each subject. Even if you think you understand a topic deeply, I encourage you to read about it, as you may either be reminded of what you already know or discover another piece of life's puzzle.

The book's first section is focused on developing your intuition and reclaiming your inner power. Here, you are encouraged to hone your intuitive skills, familiarize yourself with various aspects of your shadow, work with your energy centers, release challenging emotions and stresses from your life, and become self-empowered.

The second section urges you to master your soul's journey. You will learn to connect to your soul, access Divine Energy, open yourself to unconditional love, understand more about soul mates, work on past lives, and discover your soul purpose.

The third section is all about attracting, healing, and transforming your relationships with romantic partners, children, money, and your environment. I believe that through understanding your life, loving yourself, and embracing your soul's journey, you can live in the present moment and have a greater ability to practically handle challenges.

Finally, the last section looks at various ways of letting go of excess weight, healing heartbreak, and moving forward after loss. Here, I also encourage you to make new, empowering decisions and contemplate the possibility that death is not the end of your soul's journey.

I share many of my own experiences and stories from my clients, students, friends, and family, as I believe a story can inspire and demonstrate real-life situations in a way that theory alone cannot. Furthermore, a story can emphasize important points and stretch your mind to envision what is possible.

I would suggest that once you have read the entire book, you can feel free to work primarily with those sections that are drawing your attention.

Working with the Processes

Just as in my previous book, *The Secret Language of Your Body*, I have created processes that utilize all your senses and many aspects of your being. Feel free to combine the processes in this book with the processes from *The Secret Language of Your Body*, *The Secret Language of Color Cards*, any of my audio programs, and/or any other remedies or modalities you already utilize. I have combined a mixture of Divine connection, intention, visualization, color healing, meditation, breathing, touch, pressure-point therapy, mudras, movement, vibrational healing, sound, intention, and emotional release in the processes.

I tried to make all the processes in this book easily accessible so that you only need to spend a short time on them. As you work with the exercises, you will start to experience deep changes in yourself as well as in your life experience.

I also encourage you to keep a journal as you read the book, writing down any sections that jump out as needing work. It is also valuable to keep a record of your progress in different areas of your life.

Most processes include a clearing statement, which usually starts with a reference to Divine Intelligence. What I mean by this is Higher Wisdom, Divinity, Source, Soul, or anything that you associate with our soulful nature. If you are uncomfortable with any particular words in the processes, feel free to use your own.

At the end of each clearing statement, I ask you to repeat the word "CLEAR" to release and purify any stuck energy. In the English language, *clear* also relates to *clarity*. So the idea is to release stuckness and create clarity. For the best results, it is important that you repeat the word "CLEAR" several times, which can take between thirty seconds to a minute. Think of this as vacuum cleaning your internal house. In other languages, it is important to find an appropriate word or words that reflect this intention.

Feel free to also make up your own clearing word. And if you do, make sure the word is positive and makes you feel good when repeating it. In certain processes, I have used the words *peace*, *light*, or *surrender*. The most important thing is that you feel comfortable and can relax fully while doing the process.

How Do I Know that the Process Is Working?

When you let go of stagnation, your body might give you one of the following signs that things are releasing: tingling, yawning, slight aching, increased tension; feeling relieved, coldness, heat, more body awareness; having important insights; coughing; thirst; sleepiness; hunger; feeling more irritated or more peaceful; feeling heavier or lighter; seeing colors or bright rays; feeling warmth like a ray of sunshine; smelling a perfume; itching; sneezing; shaking; feeling dizziness, emptiness, and so forth.

Your body may also find its own unique way to give you a message that a release is occurring. You will recognize what it is when you slow down and pay attention. If you have never done any kind of healing work before, it might take you some time to release any numbness or protective barriers that you may have built up before you feel things strongly. Please be persistent and patient with yourself.

Once you do the deep work required, you will experience a huge leap in your life wellness.

Maintaining an Ongoing Practice

The greatest benefit of working with this book can be derived from practicing the processes I have included in each chapter. I have spent many years working with people, tuning in to their bodies and energy fields in order to better understand how to help them release pain, deal with distressing emotions, open their hearts, experience miraculous physical healing from disease, change their limited points of view about money, forgive their family, intensify their intuitive abilities, and connect to the Divine Source.

The processes I have included in *The Secret of Life Wellness* have been tested and refined and are now in your hands to heal, transform, and empower your life. I give you several suggestions for creating an ongoing practice. Please examine them carefully and apply them in a way that will work effectively in your life.

Through your exploration of this book and regular practice of the processes, you will intensify your intuition, connect to and work with Divine Energy, learn to clear your space, and protect yourself from dense and heavy energy. You will discover how to heal a broken heart, attract a loving partner, and experience harmony in a present relationship.

Whether you are dealing with difficult emotions, learning how to release stress, clearing your energy centers, connecting to your soul's wisdom, or in need of hope and inspiration, I encourage you to use this book as an interactive resource to help you heal, transform, and enjoy your life.

An Interactive Experience

This is not an ordinary book but an interactive experience. By using your smartphone to scan the QR codes included throughout this book, you will connect to audio links on my website where I explain certain ideas and philosophies in more detail, as well as guide you through some processes. You can discover inspiring stories, wisdom, and experiences from many people around the world who have utilized processes from this book and Visionary Intuitive Healing® seminars.

Please keep checking my website, InnaSegal.com, as I regularly add new and important information updates.

PART I

DEVELOPING YOUR INTUITION AND RECLAIMING YOUR INNER POWER

In this first section, I will help you hone your intuitive skills. After all, whether you need to heal your body, make a significant life decision, connect to an important person, safeguard your life, or find a solution to a work challenge, effective use of your intuition is a major key. As we proceed, you will reconnect with who you really are and start to see yourself and others from a softer, kinder, more loving perspective. To evolve and develop your intuitive skills, you must take time to know yourself and embrace your strengths and weaknesses.

My intention is to inspire, encourage, and demonstrate how you can simply and easily enhance, evolve, and master every area of your life, while being captivated by the exquisite design of your journey. Thus, every chapter concludes with several simple and yet profound processes, which take only minutes to do but can help you heal, transform, refine your intuition, open your heart, and embrace the various aspects of yourself.

The further you read, the more you will realize that nothing in this universe is random; every aspect of your life is designed to help you learn, grow, and expand.

1

HOW YOU CAN STRENGTHEN YOUR INTUITION

I have heard a lot about intuition and that everybody has it.
How can I strengthen my intuition and understand the difference between my
intuition and my general thoughts?

Intuition can be your guiding mechanism—your connection to the invisible, subtle, and Divine realms of existence. To be intuitive means to be able to tune in to your body, soul, or Higher Self for spiritual guidance, to decipher the messages you receive and make empowering choices. Intuitive insights can come to you when you are awake, meditating, dreaming, taking a shower, exercising, connecting to your body, or just relaxing. While you may be more likely to access your intuition when you are in a meditative state, it can arise at any point, including a time of crisis.

Mona Lisa Schulz, in her book *Awakening Intuition*, writes, "Intuition is an internal form of perception of things that are not directly in front of us in the world. It's an inner sight, a form of hearing, body sense, and emotion. It's actually common to all the other senses and an enhancement of them. What differentiates intuition from other senses is the unique form of expression it takes in each individual."[1]

The Difference between Regular Thought and Intuition

The difference between regular thoughts and intuition is the quality of information you receive. Thoughts come and go while intuition is usually a persistent feeling. Thoughts are changeable; intuition is more profound—an inner knowing. Thoughts are typically based on linear thinking; intuition is spontaneous and natural. Thoughts are fleeting, but intuition is often accompanied by bodily sensations and unexplained occurrences.

Your intuition will not necessarily give you the message you want to receive. This is one of the reasons you may tend to ignore it.

Intuition develops when you are willing to pay attention to your feelings and follow your hunches. Like exercising a muscle, the more you use your intuition, the more confidence you instill in yourself and the stronger your instincts become. The greatest power of intuitive insights is their ability to change the course of your actions and hence your life.

Your intuition awakens when you allow yourself to embrace your sensitivity, feel your emotions, and connect with nature. As you relax and allow yourself to get in touch with your body, you start to see the world around and within you from a different perspective. You begin to pay attention to messages from your body as well as the intelligence of the universe and your soul. Intuition increases when you let go of your protective barriers and open to the hidden world of wonders, where anything is possible. This is a timeless realm of guides and angelic helpers where things can transform instantly. In this nonlinear reality of Divine possibilities, nothing is bound by the rules of time, space, and gravity.

How to Recognize Intuition

Whenever I have asked my workshop participants how they recognize an intuitive insight, most have said they experience a feeling of certainty—a knowing that is often sudden, emotional, and not necessarily based on logic or prior knowledge of the details involved. They may receive an unexpected understanding, a vision, the cause of a particular issue, or the answer for what they have to do. Some also talk of feeling tingling sensations or changes in temperature, smelling scents, or experiencing a particular taste in their mouth. Others hear sounds; receive guidance through signs; or use cards, channeling, astrology, numerology, dreams, and other methods. Everyone is different and receives information in his or her unique way.

Your intuition becomes your compass, a navigating device that enhances your flexibility, adjusting your course based on internal wisdom as well as the external circumstances of your life. While I encourage you to hone your intuition throughout this book, I also believe that you need to use your intelligence, especially when making important decisions.

Most people have experienced intuitive guidance in their lives that led them to a place where they needed to be—a knowing that someone they cared about was in trouble and needed help, a sense that someone they were close to was about to pass away, or a certainty that they would get the job they wanted before they even applied. One of the greatest challenges people experience with intuition is their accurate interpretation of the information they receive.

Your Body Is Constantly Giving You Messages

In my bestselling book, *The Secret Language of Your Body*, I explore how your body intuitively communicates with you through sensations, physical pain, emotions, specific thought patterns, memories, symbols, colors, visions, tastes, smells, sounds, movements, and dreams.

Your body is constantly giving you messages about what is and is not working in your life. I have had countless friends and clients who were stuck in a difficult relationship and developed serious neck problems. Even though I would tune in to their bodies and share that it appeared that there were unresolved issues in a past or a present relationship that were affecting their neck, they would grit their teeth and tell me that all was well. Of course, as the pain became unbearable and no amount of chiropractic care helped, some were willing to start listening to their bodies, work on their emotional issues, and make life changes. It is no wonder that we have a famous saying in English that a person is a "pain in the neck." This intuitive insight has become part of our cultural way of expressing ourselves when we are having an unresolved issue with a particular person.

Intuitive Methods of Diagnosing Illness

There are many intuitive diagnostic methods. Some people can see images and cellular memories inside a person's body, tune in to energy centers, or feel other people's emotions and pain. There are also various muscle testing techniques that can assess physical, mental, energetic, and emotional issues.

I have met several art therapists and doctors who can pinpoint illnesses people have by asking patients to draw how they see themselves and how they feel about their life. Folding a sheet of paper twice to make four quarters, these doctors and therapists have the patients use colored pencils to draw and color in their face, body, family, and anything else they feel is relevant on different parts of the page. This can give an experienced health practitioner information about their patients' lives, what emotions they are dealing with, their possible aliments, and what tests may need to be done, as well as the possible causes of a patient's "dis-ease." The different quarters can also relay information about the patient's past, present, and future. This kind of intuitive drawing technique is particularly powerful with children, as it also gives them an opportunity to express themselves and understand what is going on in their lives.

Sound healing, aromatherapy, and different touch and movement treatments can pinpoint physical, emotional, and energetic problems. There are also people who use crystals, pendulums, runes, cards, or colors as tools to intuit physical, emotional, and energetic conditions. Both internal and external guidance helps to show you that you are on the right track in relation to your life purpose, as well as keeping you healthy and giving you courage to heal, evolve, and move forward.

It's important to find an intuitive system that works for you. It is also essential to remember that while intuition can help you in many areas of your life, you still need to use your common sense, have a balanced point of view, and make practical, realistic choices. Combining your intuition with wisdom and experience usually bears the greatest results.

Be careful not to become overexcited about schemes that promise magical solutions to longstanding problems. When people want an instant result, most of the time it's because they feel lost, desperate, or disempowered. From years of experience, study, and being told about people who guarantee miraculous healings, instant enlightenment, or methods to get rich quick, I have found that these solutions only work for a very low percentage of people who naturally fit the system or are able to adapt. However, most people who get involved eventually lose their power, money, time, and faith.

I always advise my clients, family, and friends to not only trust the advice that someone gives them but to also do a substantial amount of research on any conditions that they are challenged by to make informed decisions about what actions to pursue. This is particularly relevant when they have been pressured to do something that they don't understand or feel comfortable with by a doctor, health practitioner, or even an intuitive healer. For instance, I have met people who have spent a substantial amount of time doing certain breathing techniques and saying mantras without properly understanding them, literally becoming incapacitated and bedridden as they shattered different circuits in their body and nervous system. I have also known people who have spent tens of thousands of dollars on their healing, always searching for the next miracle, only to end up sicker than ever. Make sure that you research whatever system of healing you work with, ask a lot of questions, and have a profound understanding of what you are doing.

It is also important to note that healing does not always mean curing. For example, you may release an emotional issue and change your internal experience, but the physical condition will remain due to other factors. On the other hand, you may have a physical healing without changing your internal reality, in which case the problem or ailment is likely to return. If the real cause of the issue has not been dealt with, the unhealthy energy can simply move to another area of your body that is weak. Obviously, the intention is to heal on all levels and enjoy long-term well-being.

Where Intuitive Insights Come From: Internal vs. External

I believe that you have internal insights and external guidance. Internal insights occur when you become conscious of important messages or wisdom your body and soul are trying to impart about a physical problem you are dealing with, a relationship you are in, a past experience or decision that you have been hesitant about, and so forth.

You can access internal guidance through meditation or by consciously connecting to your body, or it can appear in your dreams. Pay particular attention to repetitive dreams, as the subconscious mind, soul, and intuition are trying to get your attention.

External guidance can come from the universe in the form of synchronicities, unexplained occurrences, repetitive signs, card readings, unexpected meetings, appearances of angelic beings, visions, channeling, miracles, and symbols.

Both internal and external ways give people an intuitive insight into themselves and what they need to focus on to enjoy life wellness.

Internal Guidance: Awakening Your Intuition while Meditating

When you meditate, you have the capacity to slow down your mind and connect to your body, emotions, and soul. A relaxed state is often ideal for receiving important insights. In my workshops, I always encourage people to soften their bodies, place their hands on the part of their body that has pain or discomfort, and begin their exploration by asking empowering questions, such as:

- If there were a thought pattern or a belief stored in this part of my body, what would it be?
- If there were a feeling stored here, what would it be and what situations would it relate to?
- If my body had a message for me about the actions I need to take next in order to feel better, what would it be?

You can ask any question you like. Then simply relax and allow an answer to float into your mind. The more open you are, while maintaining a clear intention of what you are asking for, the more likely you will receive an answer. When an answer is unexpected, it usually means it has come from your intuition and Higher Self rather than your conscious mind.

Internal Guidance: The Intuition of Dreams

Often, dreams can show you what you are trying to ignore, bury, and suppress. When you recognize and start to deal with hidden, shadow aspects and difficulties you are facing, your dreams usually change. Many dream analysts believe that dreams can help release unacknowledged emotions into your consciousness so that you can face a challenging issue without creating a physical ailment.

I encourage people to keep a journal of impactful dreams and intuitive insights, give themselves time to understand the dreams' meanings, acknowledge the areas they need to transform, and then take steps toward making empowering choices. In order to fully grasp what your intuition is trying to tell you, make sure you explore the shadow and the light meanings of your dreams.

Kerry's Story: A Powerful Series of Dreams

I have a friend, Kerry, who kept dreaming that her teeth were falling out. While this dream is common, it is important to interpret it based on the person's particular experience. In Kerry's case, the dream mirrored her anxiety about a long-distance relationship she was having, where she was doing all the sacrificing. Each tooth she lost in her dream represented the personal cost of her compromise. In order to be with her boyfriend, she had to put her own dreams, career, and responsibilities on hold and follow him around the world. This put an incredible financial and emotional strain on her life. She also felt like she could not be completely honest with him, thus her dream was demonstrating her loss of power, stuckness, and lack of choice.

On a physical level, teeth help you chew food and communicate. The emotional aspect of losing teeth can demonstrate feeling powerless, as well as a fear of aging and not being able to process your current experiences. Symbolically, this kind of dream shows a loss of your voice and your lack of belief in your capacity to cocreate your life experiences. It's as if you are trapped in a situation and unable to move forward. Interestingly, Kerry also dreamt of being stuck in a prison that she kept trying to escape from.

Although Kerry's intuition was clearly speaking through her dreams, demonstrating that her mind, body, and spirit felt trapped in her situation and that she was losing her strength and had to be honest with herself and her partner, she interpreted her dream to be communicating that things were getting better and that she was making positive changes. Yet from an outside perspective, she seemed to be struggling in several areas of her life, and it appeared like her soul was asking her to pay attention to what was not working in her life, be truthful, ask for support, make practical decisions, and take responsibility for her financial situation.

Through a substantial amount of self-examination and honesty, Kerry finally understood the message, shared her true feelings with her partner, made new plans for the future, felt more confident in herself, and began taking care of her financial responsibilities. Thus she really did make positive changes.

External Guidance: The Intuition of Color

Since I love color healing, I encourage people to become conscious of the role colors can play in their lives. For instance, we can tell a lot about a person's internal state by observing the colors they wear and the colors of the food they choose to eat.

At times in my seminars, I ask people to connect to a part of their body and then ask a question such as, "If there were a color in this part of your body, what would it be?" After a few moments, I inquire, "Is this a healthy color for your body? If not, what would be a healthy color?" The intention is that the message they receive will come directly from the innate wisdom of their body. The colors they see give an insight into the internal state of their body and how they can improve their well-being. I then give them a quick interpretation of the meaning of the colors and encourage them to learn about the colors they saw.

I also ask people to pick a card from my card deck, *The Secret Language of Color Cards*, which can show them what aspects of their lives they have to work on. Since everyone chooses their card without knowing what color they are picking, it is always fascinating to hear gasps of excitement when they see the color and understand how it relates to their life.

If you chose to explore color healing, I would recommend asking your body to intuitively show you what color it needs, as I have described above.

There are many different healing card decks that can give you a quick insight into something you are working on. I encourage you to surround yourself with various tools like these—tools that can help you develop your intuitive abilities.

Rhonda's Story: Color Healing

Rhonda used color healing with the help of my color cards and Reiki to assist her mother to heal her thyroid cancer. To begin the healing, Rhonda's mother intuitively chose three colors that could help with her thyroid and immune system: blue, which is helpful for any throat and thyroid conditions, as well as with purifying the body, soothing nervous irritation, and clearing blocked pathways; orange, which assists in boosting your immune system and helping to dissolve painful emotions; and green, which aids in overcoming fear, releasing frustration, and revitalizing your nervous and circulatory systems.

Rhonda then placed the cards on her mother's body and began sending healing energy to her. When she removed the cards, they had changed color and had a warm, sticky liquid on them. Her mother said she also felt like painful energy was leaving her body.

Not long after, her mother had an operation where her thyroid gland was removed. When she got her results back, they showed no cancer.

Deepak Chopra writes, "It may sound strange to think of cancer as distorted energy, but that's just what it is. To remove that discomfort, you have to start thinking of the whole body in terms of energy. Dealing with your own energy is the most effortless way to heal yourself, because you are going directly to the source."[2] I have heard of countless examples of how combining intuition with color healing and energy work can help you heal. While at times healing yourself can require deep exploration of many different aspects of your mental and emotional patterns as well as your diet and lifestyle, at other times it can occur quickly and easily. It is important that you do not underestimate the power of a simple healing process done with the right intention and an open heart.

External Guidance: The Intuition of Repetitive Signs

At times, your soul will connect to Universal Intelligence and communicate to you through recurring experiences, unexplained occurrences, and sometimes instant aid. Usually this is to assist you with shifting your perspective, healing an aspect of your life, helping someone in need, providing confidence that you are on the right track, or completely changing the course of your life. The Universal Intelligence will always try to guide you on an easier path, but if you resist, you will be impelled to grow through difficulties instead of love and joy.

Repetitive signs are the way Universal Intelligence signals to you that you are supported and not alone. It also hints that there could be a bigger picture that you are not aware of when you are caught up in fear, details, and limitations.

My Story: Following the Guidance of Repetition

A few years ago, I was teaching numerous workshops in Europe. I had several events scheduled in London, but whenever I connected to my intuition, I felt that I would not teach in London on this occasion. On a conscious level, this insight disturbed me, as I don't like canceling events, so I tried to ignore the uncomfortable sensations.

Even more unsettling was that no matter where I went, I saw huge posters inviting people to travel to Morocco. I'd never really thought of traveling to Morocco, but all of a sudden I felt an incredible and inexplicable urgency to go. Reluctantly, I canceled my trip to England and persuaded a friend to come with me to Marrakesh for four days. In Marrakesh, I greatly enjoyed visiting the sights and tasting Moroccan food.

The day before we were to return to Europe, my friend and I booked a guide to show us some spiritual sights. While we were in the car, I wondered if Marrakesh was simply an educational holiday or if there was a greater purpose to this visit. Meanwhile, my friend told our guide (who was also our driver) about my healing work.

At one point, our guide turned to look at me and asked if I knew whether doctors in Australia did eye transplants. I inquired why he asked. Without flinching, he told me of his six-year-old son, who was losing his eyesight, and that he would be more than happy to give his son one of his eyes. Touched by his unconditional love for his son, I immediately offered to go to his house at the end of the day and do some healing on his son. The tour did not end until around 10 PM, and I was exhausted. We were flying out early the next morning, but since I had offered to help, I felt it was important to keep my word.

As we walked into our guide's house, three of his young kids came out to greet us. The little boy who had problems with his eyes ran to me and gave me the biggest, warmest, most amazing hug. As I held him in my arms, I felt enlivened. This boy had something special. His energy emanated love, kindness, and wisdom. *This is an evolved soul*, I thought.

I worked with this child for more than an hour, doing every healing process I could think of that could help. But even more than that, I prayed. I prayed like I had never prayed before, with every ounce of my being. And as I prayed, I cried.

I cried because this child, who did not speak my language, moved me. I felt like he touched my soul, and as I helped him heal, I healed. I was healing my relationship with my own son. I was forgiving myself for being away from my home, for disappointing people, for being imperfect, for not being able to be in several places at once to heal all the people I wanted to help. At the same time, I felt grateful—elated even—for the opportunity to participate in healing, in giving hope, in witnessing love and miracles, in being in Marrakesh to help this one boy.

13

I taught this beautiful little boy and his parents different eye exercises and processes from *The Secret Language of Your Body* to help regenerate his eyes. When I had finished, the young boy's father talked with his son and did some eye tests, moving objects to various distances in front of his son's face. The whole family watched as the little boy was able to see at extended distances. His father looked at me with tears streaming down his face and told me that his son's vision had improved immensely. I knew that I had played a role in giving this boy and his family hope and the tools to heal.

I also understood the real purpose for my visit to Morocco.

External Guidance: Life's "Coincidences"

Sometimes we believe that we need to move in a particular direction, which seems to be the right way to proceed, and then our goals and ideas change, and the universe assists us by adjusting our path. So the messages we receive could seem contradictory; however, there are no rules in the universe that say your path should be linear instead of creative. Life is not a business meeting, which is structured, runs on time, and has clear agendas to follow.

The more you are in tune with your body and are able to develop your intuition (or as I like to call it, "internal tuition"), the more in touch with nature and the natural flow of life you will become.

It is important to note that even when you are in tune, there will be times in your life that are chaotic—when you will have doubts and feel confused. This is usually the time for internal and external change. Change often occurs on the border between chaos and order, confusion and clarity, shadow and light, fantasy and reality, success and failure, pain and pleasure. And life often challenges your flexibility, depth, and ability to adapt to these new possibilities.

Jenny's Story: Intuitive Insights with Car Accidents

My cousin Jenny was having nonstop problems with her car. In a short time, she experienced eight accidents. Jenny had been studying a course on commerce and had a job as an assistant accountant, which did not suit her personality. She felt frustrated and unhappy in her role.

One day, Jenny and I were on our way to a movie when we began talking about the messages the universe gives us. Jenny looked at me and asked if I thought that the accidents she was having could be a message. Instead of answering, I asked her to focus within and ask herself what she thought.

Her insight was that even though she had studied for five years and was glad to have learned the skills, accounting was not a suitable path for her. That night, she decided to quit her job. Amazingly, the accidents stopped and Jenny became much happier. Within days, a publicist in the company she had been working with offered her a job. Jenny found that this position fit her personality much better and opened up opportunities for travel, growth, and new ways of experiencing life.

Go to this link for more inspiring stories that demonstrate your internal and external guidance in various life circumstances.
http://innasegal.com/the-secret-of-life-wellness-downloads/inspiring-stories-demonstrating-internal-external-guidance/

Ask for Higher Help

One of the most important things we can learn is to consistently ask for higher guidance and Divine help. We do not need to wait for a crisis to seek assistance. In fact, having a daily connection and communication with the Divine realm makes your journey a lot easier, more sound, and more enjoyable.

To be truly intuitive means being able to understand and speak the language of the subtle and unseen realms. While some people are born with highly developed intuitive senses and a Divine connection, others need to take time to hone their intuitive skills.

The truth is that intuition is natural and available to all who are willing to invest the appropriate time and energy to develop it. The word *intuition* is derived from the Latin word *intueri*, the meaning of which is "to look within" or "to contemplate." I encourage you to do both. There is much hidden treasure if you dare to look.

Processes for Strengthening Your Intuition

I encourage you to regularly practice the process below, as it can help you release resistance, become more sensitive to your own wisdom, open your heart, connect to your inner power, and become more in tune with yourself and your life. There are several components of this process, so you can do them all together or pick the ones that really speak to you and practice them regularly.

Remember, to build muscle and become fit and toned, you need to exercise often. To increase your intuition, you also need to practice. Trust that you have been given the perfect instrument to receive all the help you require.

Release Resistance

Sit or stand up. Take slow deep breaths. Become aware of what you feel. Are you open and excited about receiving intuitive guidance, or are you resistant and scared? If you feel resistant, imagine holding a vacuum cleaner in your hands. Place the vacuum cleaner on the parts where you feel resistance, and imagine the vacuum cleaner sucking out all tension, fear, and conflict from your body. Keep breathing slowly and deeply while letting go of any heaviness and density in your body.

Say: "Divine Healing Intelligence, please release any resistance, tension, fear, or conflict from my body and cellular memories. Surround me with your energy of safety, support, and confidence and allow me to connect to the highest, wisest, and purest source of Divine Guidance. Thank you."

Repeat the word "CLEAR" several times, until you feel lighter.

Connect with Your Heart

When your heart is open, you are much more receptive to receiving intuitive guidance. Give yourself permission to be open. Rub your hands together for a few moments, and visualize a beautiful pink bubble of light in your hands. Allow the bubble to grow stronger, and then focus your intention of being open and sensitive to listening to your intuition. Now place your hands on your heart, and visualize the pink light moving into your heart and opening the eyes, ears, and mouth of your heart, allowing your heart to receive and communicate intuitive messages with you.

Say: "Divine Healing Intelligence, please open the ears of my heart so that it can hear the voice of my intuition; open the eyes of my heart so that it can see the truth; give my heart its voice back so that it can transmit important messages to me. Thank you."

Repeat the word "CLEAR" several times, until you feel lighter.

Work with Your Solar Plexus

The solar plexus center, located at the level of the stomach, is strongly connected to your intuition, so it is important to become aware of and release any blockages that might be stored there. Place your right hand in front of your solar plexus, facing toward your body, and move it in a clockwise or counterclockwise direction (either direction will work, as the chakra moves in both directions) with the intention of energizing and expanding your solar plexus energy center. Allow yourself to breathe slowly and deeply into your stomach area, becoming conscious of any feeling or energies that reside in your solar plexus.

Say: "Divine Healing Intelligence, please release any tension, fear, frustration, numbness, and protection that blocks me from recognizing intuitive messages from my feelings. Allow me to reconnect to, listen to, and honor the profound insights and guidance my feelings can provide. Thank you."

Repeat the word "CLEAR" several times, until you feel lighter.

Clear Stuckness from Your Ears

Your ears are constantly receiving information, which is then processed by your brain and influences your nervous system. Often, people are so affected by others that they forget to listen to themselves, and thus block this intuitive pathway.

Position your hands over your ears. If you tuned in and became aware of your ears, would they look open and clear, or would they have corks stuck in them, stopping you from listening to and hearing messages? If they look like they have corks in them, imagine taking the corks out and allowing yourself to hear intuitive messages and guidance from the highest sources of wisdom. Visualize clear, sparkling light moving through and cleansing your ears of any density, emotional armor, and stress.

Say: "Divine Healing Intelligence, please allow me to have my ears open to hearing the highest wisdom possible. Allow me to listen to my own intuition and follow its guidance. I am now willing to hear how to live my life in alignment with the universe and my highest good. Thank you."

Repeat the word "CLEAR" several times, until you feel lighter.

Open Your Third Eye

Your third eye allows you to see things beyond the ordinary realms. This is one of the gateways to owning your intuitive powers. Gently place the fingers of your right hand on the third eye, which is in the middle of your forehead. Place the fingers of your left hand at the back of your head. Imagine a bridge between these two points. Now, visualize a river of indigo light entering your third eye and moving along the bridge between these two points, clearing any stuckness, doubts, or negative patterns that could stand in your way of receiving clear images and healing messages for yourself and others. Allow any buildup of heavy energy to be released through the point you are holding at the back of your head. Repeat the process several times.

When you feel that the area is clear, imagine indigo light entering the back of your head and moving through the bridge toward the front, connecting the front and back. Observe as the light begins to shine out of your third eye. Do this several times. Imagine that this indigo light connects to the Divine Wisdom of the universe and brings messages to you that can help you and others. Give yourself permission to receive those messages.

Say: "Divine Healing Intelligence, please open my third eye with ease and grace, and allow me to see the clearest images that can assist me to heal and transform any area of my life where I am being challenged. Show me what I need to know. And where it's appropriate, assist me with helping others by showing me what they need

18

to know to help themselves. Give me the ability to see the Divine Perfection of life and how everything is connected. Open my eyes to the extraordinary opportunities that life has to offer and help me to have clear guidance. Allow me to live my life with integrity, truth, and inspiration. Thank you."

Repeat the word "CLEAR" several times, until you feel lighter.

2

HOW YOU CAN LOVE YOURSELF

I have heard people talk about loving and connecting to yourself in a deeper,
more meaningful way. At the moment, this is only a concept to me.
I would like to know how to connect to myself and those I love at a deeper level.

When my daughter, Angelina, was four years old, she said, "Mummy, I love you more than the world, more than the universe, more than all the galaxies, but I'm really, really sorry." At this point, she made a very sad face. I asked her what she was sorry about, and she said, "I love myself more." She then paused and looked at me. "Just one dot more, because it's important to love ourselves the most so that we can love other people." I was really touched and impressed by her simple wisdom.

For most people, loving themselves is an extensive journey of self-discovery, self-acceptance, and deep soul-searching. Although the words *love yourself* are commonplace in spiritual circles, not many seem to know what this means in practical terms. It is important not to reject the words but to delve deeper into their true meaning.

Overcome Obstacles to Love

Some of the biggest obstacles to self-love that I have observed are self-criticism and the need for perfectionism, which leads to harsh judgment of the self and, eventually, illness.

21

Our society teaches us to neglect ourselves and our own needs and desires. If we spend time nourishing ourselves and being soft with our imperfections, we are often told that we are weak and selfish.

I have noticed that, for many people, taking any time out for themselves is more a luxury than a daily way of life. Yet to love yourself, you must have time to connect with who you are and get to know what works for you.

Take a Journey of Self-Discovery

Instead of comparing yourself to others, discover and embrace your own strengths and weaknesses. Knowing what you love, how you want to be treated, what makes you feel safe, what food you need to eat to be healthy, what exercise you need to feel strong, what work inspires you, the space and environment you need to learn and grow are vital factors for being kind to yourself.

When you know your internal limitations, you can be more forgiving with yourself and find others who can balance your weaknesses with their strengths. They can also guide you to gently and consistently work on some of your internal restrictions so that you can grow, learn, and move forward with more freedom.

Practice the Way of Softness

From early childhood, many of us are taught to be strong, tough, judgmental, competitive, and harsh. It is little wonder that we live in a world where aggression rules. However, because we are cocreators of our own lives, we can choose to create a different reality. Our opportunity is to embrace the way of softness and kindness.

I would like you to stop reading this and take a moment to explore what it would mean to be soft with yourself this moment? When you contemplate softness, does your physiology change? Does your breath slow down? Do you feel lighter?

What does it mean to be soft and gentle with others? How would you treat others if you felt soft and peaceful in yourself? Softness and kindness can be a way of life when practiced daily.

Make Time to Connect

Loving yourself means taking care of yourself. This may involve having a time of day when you meditate, connect to your body, go for a walk in nature, do a self-healing process, read, write, play sports, meet up with friends, focus on opening and nourishing your heart.

Ask yourself: *What kind of daily experiences would help me to feel nurtured? What would make my heart sing and my spirit soar?*

Self-love can be as simple as watching a butterfly, smelling a beautiful flower, drinking your favorite drink, listening to music, playing with a child, looking in the mirror and telling yourself that you are valuable and appreciated, dancing, singing, playing sports, looking at art that inspires you, or receiving a hug from someone you love. Most important is to be in the present and to deeply appreciate the moment.

Once I started to teach people about self-healing and transformation, I saw that, in order for us to give to others, we must be able to receive love, care, and support.

If you don't currently have people in your life who envelop you with love and offer you a soft place to land when times are rough, I deeply encourage you to ask for that support in your daily meditation or prayer. And when you ask, focus on connecting to others' resonant energy and receiving them into your heart. With several of my close soul friends, my husband, and my children, I felt like I knew their spirit before we met in the physical world.

When you can give and receive love, life takes on an extra dimension. You begin to breathe, live, and emanate love. All the sharp edges of your life become smoother and you acquire the strength to keep going, even in the darkest moments.

Know Your Self-Worth

You need to know that you are worthy of the most incredible love, support, warmth, success, and happiness. Understand that, on deep subconscious and unconscious levels, you receive into your life the things you feel you deserve.

Of course, some people might read this and think, for example, "I don't deserve to be abused, yet I am." No one consciously says, "I want to be abused, poor, or taken advantage of." However, from childhood, you observe and learn what is OK through your environment, how your parents relate to you and each other, how you are treated at school, and what you are told about yourself. If you receive repetitive messages of being unlovable, unworthy, inadequate, inept, and hopeless, this is how you will feel about yourself. Unconsciously, you will create an attractor field, which will pull to you the things, people, and experiences that match your limited ideas about yourself.

Connect with Cellular Memories

As you examine your inner world, you will begin to decipher which elements are worth keeping and which beliefs, ideas, and memories you need to let go of or alter. A fascinating phenomenon I have observed is that when people discover a cellular memory, recognize it, and then slightly adjust it, their physical health and whole reality can transform.

I understand cellular memory as cells in your body storing information, memories, or traumas from earlier experiences, your ancestors, and past lives. These memories also contain information that relates to your conscious and subconscious patterns of behavior.

Stevan Thayer, founder of Integrated Energy Therapy, says, "Every cell in our body has the ability . . . to remember. Our cellular memory can store the memory of:

- Physical trauma: accidents, cuts, bruises, surgeries, or abuse
- Emotional trauma: heartache, fear, and anger
- Mental trauma: manifests as low self-esteem, feelings of unworthiness, worry

When trauma is suppressed into the cellular memory, the energy of that trauma can get stuck. The problem with suppressed cellular memory is not only does it limit our ability to live freely and joyfully in life, but it can also support the body in developing physical illness."[3]

I have guided thousands of people to connect to their bodies and consciously work with their cellular memories to heal themselves.

After many of my students got in touch with their cellular memories, they reported becoming aware of challenging past experiences that had occurred to them, even though they had rarely or never consciously thought of those events since. During the process of asking what is imprinted in their cellular memories, people have reported experiencing different bodily sensations in particular areas of their body where they have pain or discomfort, smelling fragrances, hearing sounds, seeing images, and having certain tastes in their mouth.

You may experience one or several of the above when you work with the cellular memory release process. This process helps you to let go of emotional stagnation, which can contribute to disease.

> Go to this link to work with an audio process in which I guide you to tune in to your body, release cellular memories that no longer serve you, and heal yourself.
> https://soundcloud.com/beyond-words-publishing/cellular-memories-by-inna

Susanne's Story: Working with Cellular Memories

Susanne came to see me because her knees were deteriorating at a rapid rate. She had wanted to be a writer and had recently began writing children's books. It took Susanne over five minutes to climb the steps to my office. And when she got there, she was nearly crying from pain and exhaustion. I asked Susanne to place her hands on her knees, tune in to them, and share any feelings that were stored there. Angrily, she told me she felt nothing. I gently guided Susanne to take a few deep breaths and encouraged her not to judge her feelings. She told me that she felt angry but did not want to feel this. I asked her to give herself permission to feel the anger and to discover the memory that was attached to it.

Instantly, Susanne saw herself as a seven-year-old child. She was drawing a picture and writing a few comments underneath, trying to create a little storybook. Excitedly she ran to show her mother her picture book. Her

25

mother not only brushed Susanne away but told her that her drawings were not very good. As a seven-year-old, Susanne was devastated and made a decision to stop her creative drawing and writing.

Not long after, she began experiencing slight weakness in her knees. Knees can often represent our flexibility and our ability to move forward in life. When, at fifty-seven, Susanne finally made a decision to write children's books, her knees deteriorated further. Susanne's knees were storing this memory of her childhood. When I inquired how she felt as a seven-year-old, after her mother's harsh comment, she told me she felt useless, hopeless, and worthless.

Although Susanne was following her dream of being a writer, those same feelings were resurfacing fifty years later.

I asked Susanne to slightly adjust the memory she shared. I encouraged her to imagine that a few minutes after the incident, her mother apologized for brushing Susanne away, looked at her drawing carefully, and told her that she was really proud of her and would love to see Susanne draw many more pictures.

I also asked Susanne what color would help her to dissolve the painful aspects of that memory. She said orange. Orange is a great color for clearing traumatic memories out of the cells. Susanne imagined orange light moving through her body and clearing any toxic energy that related to that particular memory. Then I asked her to visualize colors that could help her feel more confident and creative. She worked with blue, yellow, and purple.

At the end of the session, Susanne reported that her knees felt 80 percent better. She walked out of my office with more confidence to move forward.

While you cannot get rid of your cellular memories, you can make slight adjustments to them, as your subconscious mind does not know the difference between what is real and what is imagined. It is important to be aware that the newly adjusted memory needs to feel realistic to you.

Discover Your Beauty

I love Christina Aguilera's song "Beautiful." There is so much truth in the lyrics "you are beautiful no matter what they say." Although we live in an age of celebrity and beauty magazines that try to dictate to us what is beautiful and attractive and what is not, our real beauty shines from within. It is something that cannot be bought over the counter or carved by a plastic surgeon. Most of us have seen people who, while we may have looked right over them when they first entered the room, go on to light up the place and become exquisitely attractive. We no longer see their outer appearance but are enthralled by their internal radiance and light.

Part of loving yourself is seeing and cultivating your own beauty. Every time you pass a mirror, instead of judging yourself, try to see something beautiful. It can be internal or external.

Ask the people who love and care about you what is lovable and beautiful about you. And when they tell you, accept it.

Let Down Your Protective Barriers

Many people carry strong protective barriers around themselves and their hearts to shield against hurt or disappointment. But these barriers do not stop them from feeling distressed; they prevent them from opening their hearts and loving or being loved.

Self-imposed barriers impede you from using your intuition, trusting the unknown, taking chances, making powerful soul connections, diving into love, evolving spiritually, being of service, and feeling alive and joyful.

Pierre's Story: Breaking Through to Love

Pierre attended a six-day workshop I was teaching in France. He was a tall, lanky man in his early forties who seemed disillusioned by life. He told me that the only reason he came to the workshop was because he had heard me on the radio and was touched by what I said.

Pierre said that if what I taught did not work, he would abandon his search for meaning. He told me that he did not feel any emotion, see any images, or experience any connection to his body or to anyone else. In other words, Pierre was completely frozen and cut off from the wisdom of his body and soul. His skill was thinking and judging. When other people talked about having visions of something beautiful or important, Pierre said that he did not see anything. When I taught about feelings or connecting to the body, he told me he felt nothing. Most of the time, he seemed fidgety and frustrated.

After three days, Pierre came to me and told me that he'd had enough and did not think he would be coming back. I encouraged Pierre to return the following day, saying that he should wait until we finished the workshop to announce his judgment. I told him that we often have deep breakthroughs at times when we have lost all hope and expect them least. Pierre looked unconvinced but showed up the next morning. Apparently, he had forgotten something and decided he would come in the morning to fetch it.

Knowing the situation and that this was a real opportunity to transform Pierre's life and inspire others, I invited everyone to focus on themselves and ask a very important question: *Who am I?* I told the group, "If you are not your arm or leg, because if those were cut off you would still be here, and if you are not your thoughts or feelings or experiences, because they change, then *who are you*?"

The room became quiet as people began their personal exploration. After a while, I heard answers like, "I am love," "I am all there is," "I am a soul," "I am life," and so forth.

I decided to go a bit further and ask everyone to think of someone whom they had judged in the room and then look beyond their barriers and see into that person's heart and soul. Since Pierre was still resisting, I decided to tune in to him. The first thing I saw was a wall that seemed impenetrable. I intuitively asked to be shown what had created this wall. Immediately, I saw a scene of a young boy who was alone and looking for his mother to give him love, care, and attention. I knew that I was accessing a cellular memory from Pierre's childhood.

I also understood why Pierre had built up a massive fortress.

When everyone had completed the exercise, I asked Pierre to sit in the middle of the room. I looked directly into his eyes and said, "Who has hurt you so much that you have had to build a massive fortress to keep everyone out?" Pierre stared at me in shock, as if he had just been found out. Before he spoke, I told him that I wanted to hear the answer from the child part of him that had been hurt. After a few moments, Pierre whispered, "My mum."

As I had seen, when Pierre was a young boy, he desperately craved the attention of his parents, especially his mother. When he did not receive it, he felt lost, hurt, and abandoned. He made a decision that he had to be strong and need nobody. Whenever he would get close to someone, the fear of being abandoned would sweep through him, and Pierre would push that person away. In order to avoid the hurt of abandonment, Pierre numbed all his senses.

I asked one of my helpers to come into the middle of the room and to role-play with Pierre. Pierre would speak from the part of the little boy, who was holding on to the pain, and my assistant would play the role of his mother.

During the process, I saw Pierre laugh and cry until he felt more surrendered and at peace. I told him that this was his lucky day. I asked each participant to tell him what was lovable about him. As each person came up to Pierre, his face would light up and transform. I could not believe how different he looked. His face seemed open, welcoming, and soft. His whole body was vibrating, and he said that he felt like he was flying.

When this process was complete, each person in the room was touched and somehow transformed. Something deep was healing. We had a short break, and I asked everyone to sit for the next exercise, which is one of my favorites. It is one where we work on sending healing to our own and our partner's heart. The process was deep and beautiful, and I saw Pierre's face shining. When I asked him about his experience, he proceeded to tell me in detail all the things he saw and felt in his partner's heart, which she confirmed were accurate and relevant to her life. He even confessed to receiving very precise information about her past life, which she had been previously aware of. It was an extraordinary change for someone who had told me that he could not feel, see, or sense anything a few hours previously.

The next morning, Pierre, one of the first to arrive at the workshop, thanked me profusely and told me that the process we did the previous day was the most beautiful experience of his life. He asked me to wait before starting, as he had to go and pick up something special, and returned ten minutes later with two huge bouquets of stunning flowers.

I was deeply touched. What it showed me above all else is that we all need to experience love and connection. As children, we know that we are lovable, based on how our parents and people who are close to us treat us. We feel we are lovable until somehow we are told or shown that we are not.

To love ourselves, we need to be willing to know ourselves by giving ourselves time, asking deep questions, and focusing on opening our hearts. However, once our heart begins to open, we need to express this love to others as well. When we express our love, it grows and flows through our whole being.

The Magic of Love

I am extremely fortunate to have taught thousands of people to connect with their bodies and open their hearts. What I find extraordinary is when several people in a group open their hearts at the same time, as true magic happens in these moments. I have witnessed the most incredible, miraculous physical healings in the space of love: people who could hardly walk get up from their chairs and start dancing; diseases that doctors said were incurable are healed; and people let go of past baggage and fall in love with themselves, their lives, and their families. I have seen the deepest bonds created and the most fantastic opportunities open up. There have even been a few marriages.

As I write, I feel enormous gratitude for having truly experienced the energy of love. Many people write or talk about love as a nice concept. But to really open your heart—feel, touch, taste, breathe, and experience it outside the perimeters of a romantic relationship—is extraordinary. And this does not have to take away from a relationship you have with your partner but can actually enhance it.

The Healing Power of Touch

Many scientific experiments have proven that touch is healing to the human body. To love ourselves and to feel love, we need to be touched. We need to be touched on a physical, emotional, and soul level. It is so beautiful to see that more and more people are embracing the idea that hugging each other is healing.

At times, I ask people to embrace each other in some of my workshops. Often, I play a song and encourage people to hug for the duration of the song. I want people to make a real connection—to allow themselves to feel the power of touch and the strength of connecting heart to heart for several minutes.

My Story: Experiencing Oneness

Not long after I met Fred (who is part of my soul family and whom I write about in the chapter on soul mates), we agreed to catch up for dinner. We had such a powerful and pure heart connection that both of us were speechless when we saw each other. We simply could not express with words the love and gratitude we felt for having such an extraordinary and unexpected connection.

I put on some music, and for a few minutes, we sat in silence, enjoying being next to each other. I say the love was pure because our heart connection felt soulful. At one point we embraced, forgetting all about dinner. It was one of the deepest and most heartfelt hugs I have ever had. In fact, it felt like time stood still, and we were just two souls experiencing oneness.

The most incredible love flooded through every cell in my body. At one point, I could really understand what it meant to be an energy being, as nothing felt physical anymore. It was like love was vibrating through the whole room, the couch, the flowers, the walls. The experience was magnificent and unforgettable. Through it, I felt like I was healing my relationships with people, men in particular, but also my feelings about myself and the fact that I was worthy of being loved deeply, purely, and unconditionally.

You, too, are worthy of being loved deeply, purely, intimately, passionately, and unconditionally.

Processes for Loving and Connecting to Yourself

Below are three processes that can help you to connect to yourself and be more loving. They include asking questions, writing down what makes you lovable, and expanding your capacity to receive infinite love. You can do them all together or one at a time.

Connect with Yourself

In order to deepen your connection with yourself, find a place where you won't be interrupted for at least fifteen to thirty minutes. Sit up with a straight spine and take slow, deep breaths. Extend your middle and little fingers and place the others on the tip of your thumb. Do this with both hands. Focus your attention within.

Ask yourself the question, *Who am I?* Wait for an answer. Then ask the question again, this time reflecting on the following: *If I am not my body, and if I am not my thoughts, feelings, beliefs, or experiences, then who am I?* Allow yourself to explore this question while also being aware of your thoughts and the space between these thoughts.

Do this for as long as it's comfortable. Whether it is ten seconds or thirty minutes, it will be highly beneficial. This exercise will center you and allow you to begin exploring who you really are, beyond the physical, mental, and emotional aspects that you know.

You can practice this process several times a week to strengthen your connection with yourself as well as to explore the deep silence within your soul. This will also help you to feel calmer and more grounded in your everyday life.

Recognize What Makes You Lovable

To love yourself, you need to recognize all the ways that you are lovable and valuable. Take a few minutes to reflect on all the qualities that make you lovable. Write those qualities down, and place them next to your bed. Read them every day for a week. And when you read them, allow yourself to really take them in. During the week, ask all the people you care about what they love about you. Write down what they say and then focus on accepting those qualities within yourself. Really listen to what people say, and thank them for sharing what is great about you.

Once you know that you are lovable and valuable, you can begin to attract the experiences, people, and things you really desire into your life, because you will know that you deserve them.

Visualize Infinite Love

Place your hands on your heart. Close your eyes and visualize a big infinity sign on the ground. Walk the imagined line of the sign, following it with your feet. As you are walking the line of the sign, focus on everyone and everything you love in your life. Keep walking around this sign until you feel an incredible amount of love and gratitude. Then stand in the middle of the sign. Open your arms wide and imagine that the infinite love of the universe now flows into your heart. Focus on breathing this love into every cell of your body.

Now, concentrate on connecting to the people you love from a place of infinity and deep love. Give yourself permission to share your life, and communicate with them on a deep and profound level. Allow yourself to feel their love and care for you.

Say: "Divine Healing Intelligence, using the pink ray of unconditional love, sweep through my mind, body, heart, and soul and energize every aspect of my being with Divine Love. Allow me to know myself and my soul on the deepest level possible. Give me the highest, clearest, and most perfect guidance. Allow the Divine Love within me to dissolve all fear, doubt, anger, disconnection, and any other obstacle to my happiness, love, and freedom. Thank you."

Repeat the word "CLEAR" several times, until you feel lighter.

3

HOW YOU CAN EMBRACE YOUR SHADOW AND WORK WITH YOUR INNER CHILD

I heard that we have a light and a shadow side. Can you expand on this?
Also, what is a role of the inner child in our lives, and how can we work with it?

In order to regain your inner power and know and love yourself fully, it is important to understand and embrace all aspects of your light and shadow. As you study the third and fourth chapters, you will encounter the four archetypes that are part of our human makeup, including the inner child, prostitute, victim, and saboteur.

Each archetype is the keeper of many gifts and challenges, and can assist you in understanding your unconscious and subconscious patterns, behaviors, and reactions.

Working with archetypal energy can help you heal past wounds, let go of fearful and limiting patterns, release self-sabotage, reach your highest potential, reclaim your integrity, have more choices, and become self-empowered.

Embrace Your Light and Shadow

Our shadow side consists of aspects of ourselves that we are least familiar with—aspects that we bury, resist, and suppress. It is a secret hideaway where we try to mask all our insecurities, fears, disappointments, and failures, as well as our potential greatness,

35

influence, beauty, integrity, and uniqueness. We yearn to be accepted and acceptable. Often, our greatest fear is to be labeled as different, weird, or unusual. Thus, we try to detach ourselves from our deepest apprehension; that somehow we are unwanted, worthless, false, unlovable, shameful, guilty, or damaged.

In order to escape from looking within and discovering our perceived darkness, we attempt to cover up, trying our hardest to either please others or to resist them. We also project unconscious aspects of ourselves onto others. This can include positive and negative characteristics or personality traits that we disown.

We neglect to understand that our shadow aspects are the keepers of our greatest power. Much of our authenticity, potential, greatness, creativity, success, passion, and contribution in life are concealed within our own self-imposed barricades.

Since many of us are encouraged to strive for perfection, we lose sight that our true beauty, lovability, growth, and evolution arise from embracing and loving our imperfections, idiosyncrasies, and individuality.

Our ability to fully love and accept ourselves and others is greatly hindered by our need to hide and deny our limiting patterns, emotions, and behaviors. Instead of allowing our highest aspects to lead, being comfortable with ourselves, and showing others who we truly are, we hand over control of our lives to our fear, resentment, rejection, hurt, anger, and neediness, without the awareness that we are doing so. Few of us realize that our neediness can hold the gift of love and the desire to help others, just as anger can offer us passion and our selfishness can make us stop, rest, and take care of our needs.

It's amazing how many of us are as terrified to discover that we might be powerful, ingenious, and extraordinary as we are of finding out we are average, weak, or dull. Our shadow aspects become dominant when we refuse to have empathy for our own and other people's challenges.

The shadow can be viewed as painful, unprocessed parts of ourselves that have the potential to hinder many aspects of our lives at the most inappropriate moments, or when we are least prepared. As our shadow aspects are often controlled by our subconscious mind, it is easy for them to permeate our daily life and wreak chaos without us being aware of how this is occurring.

Our self-sabotage can manifest in subtle and potent ways when we arrive to places late, miss opportunities, become involved with questionable characters, misread things people say, destroy potentially empowering relationships, and so forth.

When you disown your shadow, you embark on a journey of fear, guilt, anger, and separation. You stop listening to, or trusting, the combined wisdom of your mind, body, heart, and soul and begin the process of internal confusion and conflict.

If you choose to solely follow your feelings, you can turn into an overemotional, needy, insecure, doubtful, indecisive, and dependent person. If you allow the mind to rule, you can become judgmental, controlling, and overly analytical. You are likely to make decisions based on logic and what you know without taking feelings, intuition, and wisdom into consideration. If your spiritual aspects are given all the power, you can become impractical, dreamy, and unrealistic, lost in mystical fantasies and desires of being saved. The idea is to create a healthy, balanced relationship between your heart, mind, and spirit.

As long as the mind, emotions, and soul feel split and lack the ability to communicate with each other, you will feel doubtful and unsure about what actions to take, how to connect to others, and how to live in harmony with yourself. Your shadow aspects can push you toward healing by motivating you to ask questions and embrace more of who you are.

In order for you to become self-empowered, you need to move from living outside yourself to connecting to your body, intuition, and inner life. This requires bringing light to those shadow aspects that are entrenched in limiting patterns and helping them to mature.

For example, you may be repressing the fact that you are not emotionally and energetically compatible with your partner. If you were honest, you would confront your partner and work together on changing your relationship, or you would choose to leave the relationship. This would require courage, trust, candor, and a lot of personal growth. However, if you were to keep suppressing the fact that your relationship is not working, because you are afraid of being alone, you might become negative and aggressive, lie, cheat, or cause destruction in your life, creating dis-ease just to be safe.

A huge part of your healing journey is to confront your shadow aspect, take back your power—your life force energy—and expand your freedom and the choices available to you.

Colin's Story: Confronting the Shadow

Colin, a successful businessman, was married with four children. When Colin first called me for a distance healing, he was extremely secretive and protective. While I was tuning in to him, I received an image of a frog who was trying to pass himself off as a prince. (I often see archetypal images that help me to understand what is really going on in a person's life.)

I had a strong impression that he was dishonest and destructive in his life. After a little prodding, I discovered that Colin was trying to be a savior to women who had been abused and who were often deeply unhappy.

His mother had experienced severe abuse from his father and had lost several members of her family in her youth. As a child, Colin stood helplessly by her side, watching her suffer. By trying to help the women who showed up in his adult life, Colin was trying to save his mother. The problem was that these women were becoming attached to him and draining him of all his energy. Colin's pattern resulted in him neglecting his family, lying to his wife, and entering into sexual relationships with the women he'd tried to help. It was like Colin was living two separate lives but was not present in either. However, the risk gave him such a high that he felt addicted.

I saw that Colin was walking on the cliff's edge. He was gaining weight, feeling heavy and powerless, and losing his energy and concentration. He was risking his family and his life. Although it was difficult, Colin was willing to confront his shadow and deal with his challenging childhood. We discovered that besides the savior archetype, he also had a rebel inner child who loved risk. "The bigger the danger, the higher the thrill" was his motto. Although the lighter aspect of the rebel child had allowed Colin to become successful, confident, and make 50-million-dollar deals, the shadow side was seducing women and being seduced, lying, hiding, and living a double life.

Colin realized he was close to losing his family and possibly his life. He began exploring his childhood, working with his inner child and learning about his ancestry. Colin realized that if he did not deal with the patterns he'd picked up from his parents, he would pass them on to his children.

Although his mother had died, Colin spoke to her spirit and found peace. He then understood that his dad's selfishness and cruelty came from the lack of love he felt from his father. As Colin healed his past, he was also able to heal his present, stop lying and cheating, and open his heart to his family. He lost weight, left the corporate world, set up his own business, and began meditating and connecting to his inner strength. Colin's willingness to understand and work with his inner child changed his life.

The Archetype of the Inner Child

An archetype is a universally understood aspect of a personality trait, psychological pattern, or behavior. Archetypes come from mythology and are part of our universal psyche. Thus, they have a huge and active influence on our lives. The major role of an archetype is to alert you to potentially destructive patterns within your psyche and to aid you in transforming them into healthy and empowering points of view, feelings, and behaviors.

Many of your childhood beliefs, occurrences, points of view, unprocessed energies, and emotions are held within your inner-child archetype. This archetype is concerned with family, support, care, and security. When dealing with the shadow aspects of this child, you must help it to find safety and comfort in change, allowing it to understand that transformation can be energizing and fun, and can bring about new and exciting opportunities.

Much of the anxiety that people experience is related to their childhood and the aspect of their inner child that felt unsafe, vulnerable, and powerless to change things.

If, as a child, you had to take on too much responsibility for your family and grow up too fast, it is possible that aspects of your mental, emotional, and spiritual maturity were stunted.

As an adult, you may suffer, feeling like you never had a chance to experience the innocence, freedom, hopes, dreams, and inventiveness of a child. You may feel burdened by responsibilities, and sabotage your relationships and career because you want to experience more fun. You may abandon your responsibilities, get lost in fantasies, demand attention, or need someone to take care of you. On a physical level, you may feel depressed, heavy, and unwell. Many digestive conditions, kidney problems, chronic lower back pain, and fertility problems are related to the inner child's inability to process his or her childhood pain. To feel healthy and balanced, you may need to work with your abandoned inner child—help it to feel loved and accepted—which will lead to its growth and evolution.

Some of the strongest desires your inner child has is to be acknowledged and nurtured. It holds much of your creative, spontaneous, and mystical potential. When you are in tune with your inner child, it can literally magnetize magical experiences, attracting events that seem Divinely inspired and synchronistic. On the other hand, if you deny your inner child, it can plague you with doubts, fears, and insecurities, preventing you from moving forward and achieving success.

The inner child holds both personal and universal patterns, and behaviors of a particular aspect of a person's energy.

Although you may have never been physically abandoned as a child, at a particular moment in your life you may feel drawn to the abandoned child archetype, such as a time when you might be going through a difficult breakup. Working with this archetype can heal feelings of rejection, isolation, loneliness, and misunderstanding that you have carried throughout your life.

When you work with the inner child archetype, you become softer and gentler. You begin to understand that this archetypal energy is there to help you. It can assist you to heal past wounds and embrace joy, lightness—a sense of adventure, fun, and spontaneity.

When you become conscious of this archetype, you gain awareness of how it operates in your life, and if it serves you or not. When you accept and embrace your inner child, it creates support, wisdom, and healing in all areas of your life, rather than cre-at-ing chaos and destruction.

Aspects of the Inner Child

Often, people can relate to different aspects of the inner child at particular times in their lives. Through working with thousands of people, I have observed four common types of inner-child archetypes: the abandoned, the wounded, the rebellious, and the Divine. Below, I have tried to share brief explanations about them.

Before we dive in, remember that due to the fact that every psyche is individual, the inner child can present itself in a myriad of ways. If you feel drawn to delve deeper, you may discover more archetypes, such as the nature child, the dependent child, and the eternal child, amongst others. It is important, however, to not get caught up in labels, as these are just general examples that can be beneficial to explore.

(Note: For the ease of writing, I will call the inner child "it" instead of "he or she.")

The Abandoned Child

The abandoned inner child feels unaccepted, undervalued, and misunderstood. It does not feel a sense of belonging and often experiences feelings of loneliness, isolation, and rejection. The abandoned child seeks constant approval, and experiences confusion and self-doubt. It can struggle with the concept of growing up and taking on responsibilities.

On the lighter side, through support and healing, the abandoned child can claim its independence, courage, and self-empowerment. It will then connect to others from the heart, and demonstrate compassion and understanding in challenging situations. The abandoned child will then feel liberated and creative, and play with others without fear of being hurt.

The Wounded Child

The wounded inner child feels hurt, neglected, and mistreated. It experiences feelings of victimhood, violation, and trauma. It is easy for the wounded child to blame others and to see the world as a scary, difficult, painful place. The wounded child often experiences dysfunction in close relationships with others.

On the lighter side, the wounded child has an opportunity to learn compassion, forgiveness, and self-empowerment. Often, through its own healing, the wounded child develops a desire to be of service and assistance to others, helping others to grow, expand, and experience love and healing.

The Rebellious Child

The rebellious inner child resists control and order, and therefore experiences difficulties fitting into society, systems, situations, or the set of rules it has been given. The rebellious child feels limited, bored, and tired of conforming.

It is easy for the rebellious child to push boundaries, demand change, disregard others' beliefs, and get into trouble. The rebel can be blasé about potentially dangerous situations, start uprisings, break the law, lie, take advantage of and abuse others, take drugs, gamble, and generally reject authority.

The lighter, softer side of the rebellious child sees the limitations that are presented and refuses to buy into them. It can be an explorer, dreamer, and innovator. Creativity is the forte of the rebellious child, who often disregards boundaries and moves mountains to make its dreams a reality. The rebel can assist others to let go of old, outdated ideas and introduce them to a more innovative way of living.

The Divine Child

The shadow of the Divine child emerges when there is loss of hope, and the possibilities of life and the magic are not readily apparent. This can manifest as depression, fatigue, and lethargy. Under its shadow, this child, who was once an adventurer and saw the potential in everything, no longer believes that life is worthwhile, or that there is a possibility of achieving its dreams.

On the lighter side, the Divine child believes that miracles and blessings are not only possible but everyone's Divine right. This child is full of creativity, inspiration, and wonderful ideas. Life seems like a magical playground. The Divine child believes in higher intelligence and connects easily to Divine Love and Wisdom.

Working with the Inner Child

You can work with the inner child in many ways. You can do visualization exercises, for example, where you relax and imagine a child aspect of yourself. Ask this child questions about how it feels, what it believes, what hurts it, what makes it happy, how you can support it, as well as: *What do you need to heal, feel nurtured, be healthy, and to grow?*

Inner-child work is very powerful and something you need to do regularly. As you work with your inner child on all its different beliefs about your parents, money, jobs, and relationships, you will see how all these things shift in your life. You will also be able to sense a happier, healthier inner child. As your inner child is linked to your sacral energy center, you will find that this center becomes stronger and more vibrant. And because this center is connected to your ability to manifest things into physical reality, you will also find that your creative abilities strengthen and that you are able to manifest more of what you desire in your life.

Many people who have been ill have benefited greatly from working with their inner child. Often, by healing aspects of themselves that were desperately searching for love and nurturing, their health problems dramatically improved or completely disappeared.

Several clients have also told me that their relationships with their children, parents, and partners improved dramatically after they worked with their inner child. They reported an increase in confidence, inner strength, and love. Some of my clients even lost large amounts of weight after realizing that they were carrying it to protect their inner child.

My Grandfather's Story: Healing His Inner Child

As a child, my maternal grandfather, Misha, developed a rare kind of courage, intuition, and survival instinct. He demonstrated audacity that left his older siblings and their friends in awe. Unfortunately, at the tender age of fourteen, he was unjustly captured and cruelly punished for something he did not do: One day, while walking home, he noticed a crowd of people in heated discussion. Curious, he approached them and noticed a broken lock on the ground. Someone had broken into a local bakery and stolen some bread. Just as Misha was discovering what had happened, a swarm of policemen arrived, grabbing everyone who was in the vicinity of the bakery.

Misha was falsely convicted and sentenced to ten years at a labor camp in Siberia. The conditions were ghastly, and very few survived the harsh labor, starvation, bitter cold, cruel beatings, and random killings. Instinctively, Misha used the power of his mind, his intuition, and a strong resolve to endure the brutal years until his release. Incredibly, as an adult, he was strong, loving, gentle, and fearless. The deeper scars of his torturous experiences began to emerge more obviously as he progressed into his seventies.

Several years ago, I was exploring the power of ancestral memories and their profound effects on family lineages. I knew that neither of my grandparents had done much healing of their traumatic childhoods. (For many years in Russia, speaking aloud about your suffering during the war or in camps could put you at risk of going to jail or being killed.) Their only release was sharing their experiences fifty years later.

Through my own work on myself, as well as on people in my immediate family, I knew that my grandparents' traumas had been passed on. For instance, during my teenage years and early twenties, I had a strange but deep fear of being homeless. For a long time, I could not understand where it came from. One day, I was talking to my cousin, and she shared that she experienced the same anxiety. I realized then that both of my grandparents were homeless during their teens and early twenties. Their unprocessed distress was passed on to us, even though neither my cousin nor I ever had a real reason to fear homelessness. Once I recognized where this anxiety was coming from, I was able to release it and help my cousin.

On a particular visit to my grandparents' apartment when my grandfather was already nearing eighty, we began discussing his childhood. During this time, I was having a lot of difficulty communicating with him, as he was extremely pessimistic. It got to a point where I would avoid asking him how he was feeling to escape an onslaught of negativity.

However, this day was different. He shared his experience of spending ten years in a labor camp in a profound and touching manner. At one point, I could feel the deep sadness welling up in my chest and throat. As tears began to roll down my face, both my grandparents, who had difficulty expressing sadness, told me that I should not be upset about something that happened more than sixty years ago.

To avoid making them uncomfortable, I quickly told them that I had to leave. I then got into my car and drove, fighting the tears that would not stop streaming down my face. When I arrived home, I began to cry uncontrollably. It was like I was weeping from the depth of my soul. At the same time, I had a funny feeling that I was not sobbing for myself.

Since I had heard my grandfather's story several times before, I couldn't understand why I was feeling so devastated. Then in my mind's eye, I saw an image of my grandfather's inner child. He appeared to me like a malnourished, wounded fourteen-year-old boy. I saw him as clearly as if he were standing in front of me.

I closed my eyes and envisaged gently holding and comforting him. My grandfather's inner child intuitively conveyed that when he found out he had to go to Siberia, he was extremely distressed. He didn't know if he was going to his death, or if he would ever see his family again. He also shared that he had convinced himself to be strong and do anything he could to survive. Thus, he never cried or allowed himself to feel weak. I told him that if he couldn't cry, I would cry for him.

I sobbed for more than an hour, after which I felt completely cleansed and clear. My grandfather's inner child also looked better, healthier, cleaner, and more relaxed. He then started to grow, thanked me, and merged with my adult grandfather.

After that, as if by magic, my grandfather changed completely. He became positive, upbeat, and optimistic. When I called to inquire how he was feeling, he told me he felt great, he joked and encouraged me to visit. It was like the dark, heavy, depressed energy he was carrying had lifted. Everyone in the family noticed his incredible transformation, which lasted until my grandmother's death.

This experience showed me that sometimes people who are close to us are unable to work with their inner child, or unconscious issues, and that there are moments when we are able to help—even from a distance.

Finances and Your Inner Child

It is interesting to note that many people who have deep financial challenges may be operating their business or work life from the perspective of an inner child. This can occur because that aspect can feel more comfortable with receiving a limited allowance, rather than an abundant salary. You may have also observed how your parents dealt with money and then created situations in your life that either mirrored their experience or rebelled against how they would act.

Jade's Story: Money and the Inner Child

Jade, in her fifties and quite distressed about her financial situation, contacted me for a healing session. A health professional herself, Jade had a pattern of earning just enough to "make ends meet" and was always struggling with money no matter how hard she worked.

When I tuned in to Jade's energy, I saw that her inner child was throwing money out of her hands. Jade admitted that whenever money came to her, she could not hold on to it.

I guided Jade to visualize her inner child, talk to her, and ask why she was throwing money away. Her inner child answered that when Jade was young, her father, who was very successful with money, was never home. She saw her father as being lonely and unhappy. Jade associated money with unhappiness, which she didn't want to create in her life.

After explaining this to her inner child and working with her through meditation, writing, and visualization, Jade's situation changed dramatically. Within a week of doing this process, money and abundance began to flood into her life. Within six months, she had achieved several of her major goals. A year later she opened her own school of alternative medicine. She said it was like everything had suddenly become easy, and whatever she asked for started to flow into her life. Her inner child began working with her rather than against her.

Processes for Healing Your Inner Child

Working with and learning how to heal your inner child can transform your life, allowing you to make empowering decisions with the help of your present wisdom as well as the creativity, joy, and enthusiasm of your inner child.

Connect to Yourself as a Newborn

If you have a photo of yourself as a baby, find the photo and look at it. What do you feel when you look at this photo? Close your eyes and imagine holding yourself as a baby in your arms. How do you feel about yourself as a baby? Do you feel loving and nurturing or cold and blasé? How do you, as the baby, feel about your life? Are you excited or fearful? If the baby had a voice, what would the baby say? Listen as you take slow and deep breaths. Then send some loving, caring, supportive energy to help the baby feel safe and confident. Imagine the baby surrounded by a soft, pink light. Then allow it to merge with you.

Write a Letter to Your Inner Child

Become aware of the inner-child archetype you relate to the most. If you can, find a photo of yourself when you were a child that reminds you of the aspect you have chosen to focus on. If not, visualize it.

Take a pen and paper, and write down why you feel a strong connection to this aspect of your inner child. You can also write a letter to yourself from this aspect of your inner child, honestly sharing all your feelings without any restrictions or judgments from your older, responsible self.

Allow the child to tell you how it felt about your parents, siblings, friends, and teachers when you were a child. What did you need to say when you were a child that you could not say? Give the child permission to share honestly.

Then write a loving and honest response from yourself as you are now.

Ask your inner child what it needs to be happy and healthy, and then keep giving those things to it. If what your inner child has to share with you in the letter is quite negative, then I suggest that you burn the letter. Visualize being loving and caring with your inner child. Give it the love and the attention that you may have never gotten from your parents. Make a commitment to regularly communicate with your inner child and nurture it.

If you would like to do further work with your inner child, you may wish to purchase the "Healing Your Inner Child" audio program from InnaSegal.com.

4

How You Can Understand and Work with Your Major Archetypes

I've heard that every person has several archetypes that they can work with;
however, there are four major ones that everyone has.
What are they, and how can we understand them better?

The study of archetypal aspects and influences is an in-depth exploration. There are many excellent books and workshops that give people a comprehensive understanding of these energies. I have already touched on the inner child and how it can influence our lives. The other three archetypes that are part of each person's makeup are the prostitute, the victim, and the saboteur. Each archetype presents you with important lessons and gifts, and reveals your ability to exercise your power—or lack of it—in many crucial areas of your life. It is important to understand archetypal patterns because they help you delve deeper into your subconscious and unconscious thoughts, your emotions, your energies, and your behaviors.

As discussed in chapter 3, every archetype has two components: the shadow and the light. The shadow shows us the parts that are buried deep within, occupy our subconscious mind, and often emerge unexpectedly, in destructive ways. The light aspects show us the opportunities to reach our highest potential and to live from a place of gentleness, integrity, and power.

49

Energy Centers and the Four Archetypes

Through many years of exploration, I have discovered that each of our four major archetypes have an important relationship with a particular energy center. For instance, the prostitute archetype is connected to the first energy center, also known as the root chakra; the inner child to the sacral; the victim to the solar plexus; and the saboteur to the heart center.

This means that whenever you work with a particular archetype, you help clear that center as well as heal other organs and aspects of your life that the archetype relates to. And when you release patterns from an energy center that connect to a specific archetype, you will empower that archetype and bring more confidence and clarity to your life.

The Prostitute Archetype

The prostitute archetype is connected to your fears around survival. It helps you learn lessons in relation to your integrity and inner strength. It asks questions such as, *Are you willing to sell your spirit, your loyalty, your body, or your morals for money and physical survival, or do you have the courage and the stamina to stand up for what you believe in and do what you love?* This can be particularly challenging if you are part of a family that has specific expectations and beliefs about what career you should be in, who you should marry, and how you should live your life.

This archetype also examines your faith and sincerity. It prods: *Are you willing to be honest with yourself and others, or would you rather pretend, lie, and take advantage of people in order to survive or to get ahead?* Through exploring the prostitute archetype, you must decide if you are going to live your life based on fear and the temptation to seduce, control, and sell out, or if you are going to live with love, Divine Guidance, faith, and self-worth. A question you need to consider: what is the price that you are willing to put on your physical security?

Whenever you take a step on your path of self-empowerment, you are likely to encounter someone who will want to test your inner strength by exploiting, manipulating, and taking advantage of you in order to make themselves more powerful. While your shadow prostitute may urge you to give up your honor, creativity, joy, and freedom of thought, the light aspect can help you to keep your power and your integrity, and to stand your ground.

Shadow Prostitute

Humans are known for trying to find shortcuts to everything from financial success to empowerment, healing, evolution, and love. We live in a society of instant gratification, and the shadow prostitute is constantly asking: *What is in it for me? What more can I get from this experience? How can I make others feel that I am more important, intelligent, successful, evolved, interesting, and powerful than I really am? How can I make others look up to me and want me, because I am attractive, have special abilities, important connections, money* . . . and so forth.

The prostitute archetype demonstrates the difference between self-imprisonment, dishonesty, domination and freedom, self-expression, and self-empowerment. It gives you a choice to use your power, talents, and abilities for the positive or the negative. If you believe that you are Divinely guided and put your trust in the higher powers, then this archetype makes it more difficult for you to be controlled, manipulated, or bought.

Embracing the Prostitute

When you embrace the prostitute archetype, it can be your biggest ally. It can forewarn you when you consider acting out of integrity in order to gain something in the physical. It can also infuse you with the courage and the perseverance you need to follow your heart.

When you move away from the situations and the people who use you, and cost you too much energy, time, emotion, and dignity, you can truly heal and transform your life.

Linda's Story: Befriending Her Prostitute Archetype

Many people prostitute themselves by staying in abusive relationships or in jobs they hate. Due to habit and fear, they remain in a toxic environment, disregard their principles, and make themselves ill to ensure their financial security and status—rather than change, take responsibility, and grow.

Linda had been married to her husband for over twenty years. They ran a successful business together and had three children. Although her relationship looked outwardly perfect, Linda was deteriorating inside. Every year, she would have a new health condition and part of her body would degenerate. Linda had her thyroid taken out, cysts in her breasts, problems with her ovaries, heart palpitations, back pain, toenail fungus, and migraines. Her body was screaming out, but she kept finding excuses to stay in an unhealthy relationship rather than leave it. The turning point came when she was lying in the hospital being checked for a brain tumor.

Although her physical security was important, Linda decided that being honest with herself and staying alive was essential. So at fifty-two, Linda left her husband. She moved out within a week and began a journey of self-inquiry.

Although people thought that Linda was completely insane to leave her husband at her age, and with such a small amount of money and low job prospects, deep inside Linda knew that the relationship she had with her husband was unhealthy and their journey was complete. She felt she had always hid behind him; the relationship was unbalanced and often abusive, and it was killing her. She had always stayed for the sake of security, the children, and to avoid trouble, but her children had grown up and, in a sense, it was time for her to as well.

Linda knew that her first step was to heal and listen to the wisdom of her body. She learned about archetypes, and began to work with and understand the challenges—and the power—of the prostitute. In particular, she felt she had to own the part of herself she called the "bad girl."

As Linda felt stronger, she joined a dance class. This helped her to get fit, flexible, and creative. It inspired her to open a shop with a spiritual twist and to organize healing and dance workshops that gave people an opportunity to learn about themselves and regain their inner power.

Although it took time, Linda's health improved, she met a lot of interesting people, and she made new friends. Inside, she felt alive and valued. She also learned to receive support and find creative ways to deal with challenging situations.

Linda had to befriend and listen to her prostitute archetype in order to heal. She said that she could not have imagined consciously working with the prostitute energy until she left her husband, as it would have been too confrontational. However, having a profound relationship with this archetype gave Linda the courage to follow her dreams, keep her integrity, and find a strong life purpose.

The Victim Archetype

You may become conscious of your inner victim when you experience rejection, violation, injustice, inequality, prejudice, and blame for things you did not do.

As most people experience many challenging situations throughout their lives, it is easy to qualify for a place in the victim club. The victim club contains many people who blame others, the government, society, their bodies, and their economic situation for not having what they need or desire. It is easy to point a finger at someone else, but to take responsibility for your actions, beliefs, and the roles you play in the victim drama is much more difficult, requiring you to grow, change your perspective, be courageous, and stand up for yourself and what you believe in.

It can be easy to allow the victim to take over when you feel that life is unfair. The victim can keep you safe, making you judge others superficially, holding on to past pain, or dealing with life destructively. You may feel unhappy in your current situation but comfortable with what you know. The victim can precipitate your fears and give you a list of reasons to remain the same.

Shadow Victim

When someone is in the victim state, they feel vulnerable, weak, and defeated. They are unable to stand up for themselves and create healthy boundaries. The victim enjoys getting sympathy from as many people as possible. Energetically, the victim drains whoever it is around and often finds reasons why nothing is going to work, why they will fail, or why they will end up in an unpleasant situation.

The shadow victim often avoids conflict or confrontation but feels comfortable gossiping and speaking negatively behind people's backs. This archetype also perpetuates the belief that that life is too hard, that there is no point in trying, and that if you give things a go, you might end up alone and worse off than before. The victim makes you feel sorry for yourself, for trying the path of healing and transformation, and for moving away from everything you know even though it may be harming you.

Embracing the Victim

The light side of the victim is the victorious part that helps you take responsibility for your reactions and gives you the courage to take positive actions in challenging situations.

Through this archetype, you begin to understand your relationship with power, courage, self-worth, personal boundaries, honesty, endurance, and self-respect. As the victim often arises in personal relationships, the light side can teach you to hold your power without getting angry, nasty, or vicious with others.

People can misinterpret empowerment as aggression. However, genuine empowerment is about connecting to your intuition and acting from a place of wisdom and compassion. The victorious part encourages you to heal past hurts and see them as opportunities to grow and become stronger.

Stacey's Story: Accepting the Victim

Stacey was a very successful stylist. In fact, she worked with the rich and famous, helping them look great! After twenty years in the industry, Stacey felt that her life was out of control and decided to take a break. However, deep inside, she felt like a victim, and without a job, living alone in a big city, and about to turn fifty, she found herself feeling miserable and useless.

Stacey's parents lived in a different state, and she had not spoken with them in years, as she blamed them for a lot of the pain she had endured.

Stacey's only daughter lived overseas, and they had limited contact. Stacey joined yoga classes and signed up for personal development workshops in order to get her confidence back, but she didn't feel better, as her inner victim was too strong.

When she discovered there were no quick fixes, Stacey became angry, judgmental, jealous, and spiteful. She alienated all her friends by making nasty comments and pushing them away whenever they tried to help. In fact, she proclaimed that she was taking back her power, while in reality, she was disempowering herself and using anger to protect herself from feeling vulnerable and receiving help.

In her mind, Stacey told herself that she was better than everyone else. However, in reality, she felt depressed and useless. Her body was reacting through allergies, food intolerances, and eventually an autoimmune disease.

After spending a lot of time alone, Stacey realized that although it was difficult for her to admit it, she was acting like a victim. The more Stacey explored her shadow side and owned the victim aspect of herself, the more alive she felt. She understood that her patterns were coming from her family line—her mother and grandmother in particular. She also felt angry about how women had been treated for many centuries and was directing this energy against the men in her life.

Stacey decided that she would be gentler with herself, and that she needed time to process what was stored in her body and mind so that she could truly transform. She spent several years working with the shadow and light aspects of herself, forgave her family, and slowly improved her relationships with them. Eventually, Stacey went on a six-month trip with her daughter, where they reconnected, had fun, and shared new perspectives on life. While traveling, Stacey also met Christopher, a wonderful man who practiced Tibetan medicine and helped her heal her body and open her heart.

Although Stacey no longer felt like a victim, she knew that she had to be aware that her victim archetype would continue to show her areas in her life where she had difficulty taking responsibility or felt hurt. She also recognized that this archetype could help her grow in her relationship with Christopher and others.

The Saboteur Archetype

The saboteur can cause you to sabotage opportunities, resist healthy and enriching relationships, close your heart, and lose money. This archetype is linked to your fears of surviving in physical reality. It can plague you with doubts of not being able to pay your bills, fit into society, find the right job, or have the relationship of your dreams.

The saboteur is most fearful of change, especially if that change is going to rearrange your whole reality. However, if you invest in strengthening your soul rather than sabotaging tactics, the saboteur will assist you to become more resilient and courageous.

As the saboteur archetype is connected to the heart center, it plays a significant role in your intimate relationships as well as your innermost hopes and dreams.

When you befriend the saboteur, you become acutely aware of its sabotaging tactics and how to minimize them. This gives you an opportunity to take chances and become courageous, daring, creative, and adventurous—without compromising personal responsibility. Your intuition and ability to listen to your heart's wisdom also greatly increases, and you become aware of the difference between fear, excitement, desire, and true gut instinct.

Shadow Saboteur

On the shadow side, the saboteur can guard your heart and push away any people or opportunities that make you joyful. It is a master at making up dramatic stories that have little to do with reality but cause you to doubt your instincts. It urges you to give up or postpone your dreams for fear that you are not good enough and will fail.

Whenever you try to get too close to people, the saboteur will help you to subconsciously create situations that cause conflict and pain, and leave you feeling disappointed, hopeless, or lonely. It can also judge, criticize, and put you down, telling you that you are unworthy of good things. Thus, you may stop trusting the wisdom of your heart without realizing that the saboteur is running the show. The role of the saboteur is to protect you. What it does not realize is that by trying to shield you from pain, it actually perpetuates it.

Embracing Your Saboteur

Once you confront your saboteur and understand how it is trying to keep you safe, you can develop a healthy relationship with it. Instead of creating pain, it can alert you to wonderful opportunities and lead you toward acceptance, forgiveness, self-love, and joy! It can also show you all the choices that are available to you, help you overcome your fears, and reclaim the courage you need to live your life from a space of love.

Kevin's Story: Opening the Heart

Kevin, in his early forties, worked in finance and had not been in a relationship for five years. He came to see me because he had problems with blood pressure. After helping him release a lot of stress and change his lifestyle, he was ready to tackle his issues around relationships.

Kevin had a very challenging relationship with his mother and saw an aspect of his mother in every woman he met. I asked Kevin to share ten reasons why it could be positive to open his heart to love. Instead, he told me twenty reasons why it would be better to keep his heart closed.

I encouraged Kevin to attend some workshops where we did a lot of intense heart work. He agreed, but showed up late with a runny nose. He told me he almost did not attend, as his body passionately resisted connecting to his heart.

I understood that he was scared to change and allowed his saboteur to run his life. During the heart-opening process, however, he let go of the shield he'd carried around in his heart for many years. By the end of the day, Kevin looked different. He told me that for the first time in years, his heart had opened and he was receptive to someone he could share a loving relationship with.

I saw Kevin for a healing session a few months later, and I could not believe how he had transformed. There was a sparkle in his eyes, he had changed his hair and his clothes, and most of all, he looked lively. There was also an ease about him, which I had never seen. I had a strong feeling that he had found someone. In fact, he commenced a relationship with a woman I had known for many years, who had also attended some of my workshops. They have been together for many years since and have a beautiful, nurturing relationship.

Processes for Working with Your Archetypal Energy

Below are two processes that can help you work with your archetypes and transform your relationship with them.

Move with Your Prostitute Energy

When working with the prostitute energy, connect with your first energy center, also known as the root chakra. The dominant color of the root chakra is red, and it is located around the lower hips and genital area.

While standing, place your hands on your hips and take three slow, deep breaths. Put on some music with tribal beats and shake your hips. As you shake, feel your connection to your body.

Imagine inviting the prostitute energy into your space. Visualize it as someone who is part of your circle of friends. Ask it to show you, through dance, how it affects your life. In other words, does it lead or follow, and is it supportive or disruptive in its role? Do you live your life from a place of listening to yourself and doing things because you believe in them, or do you take action primarily out of the need for money, through fear, and because it's easier not to question aspects of your life and remain the same?

Imagine that you could talk to this part. Stop moving, sit, or lie down and relax your body. Ask your prostitute archetype some questions in an attempt to get to know it better. How does it help you? How does it harm you? How can you use its passion, power, and strength to transform your life?

Don't worry if you don't get all the answers the first time you begin exploring this aspect of yourself. As you connect to your own wisdom and ask questions, you will start to receive answers and be guided to people who can support you.

Meditate for Change

Sit with a straight spine. Take some deep breaths. Make a fist with the fingers of both hands. Place your fists just above your belly button, with both your fists and the thumbs touching.

Imagine that there is a red fire burning in front of you. As you focus on the red flames, reflect on where in your life you are being dishonest and prostituting yourself. As you breathe in, imagine that the red flame moves inside your body and begins to dissolve any fear of change. Then visualize breathing in a blue ray of courage and faith. Give yourself permission to listen to the light side of the prostitute energy that can help you do what you love and be a success. Take your time with this process.

Next, imagine that the victim aspect of you comes and sits by the fire. Without words, it shows you moments in your life where you felt and behaved like a victim. It also gives you an insight into the choices you made based on a victim point of view and the consequences of those choices.

Now imagine a huge television screen materializing in front of you. A different aspect appears—one that looks a little like the victim, except it is confident, clear, and fearless. This is the victorious part of you. It turns on the television and shows you some potential futures you may experience if you choose to live your life from an empowered perspective.

Place your hands on your heart. Become aware of the ways you shield and protect your heart.

Imagine that your saboteur aspect stands next to you. It tells you that it is the guardian of your heart: it can either keep your heart closed to people and expansive opportunities, or it can open your heart while still offering the wisdom of experience—

so that you do not sabotage further opportunities for growth, love, and happiness. It also holds aspects of your heart that you have disowned. This includes the ability to love, laugh, have fun, and listen to your heart's wisdom. Allow yourself to take these abilities back.

Imagine a huge, bright, pink energy of love flowing into your heart, cleansing and energizing it. Now, visualize a yellow light of fun and laughter dancing around your chest and making you feel lighter and happier. Be aware of any other images and feelings that come to you.

Say: "Divine Wisdom, allow my healing and transformation to occur with ease, grace, and softness. Help me to receive the wisdom from my archetypes, and assist me to befriend them. Allow me to have patience and compassion with myself and others, and to evolve at the right time and in the right pace. Thank you."

Repeat the word "CLEAR" several times, until you feel lighter.

5

HOW YOU CAN USE YOUR ENERGY CENTERS TO HEAL AND SPIRITUALLY EVOLVE

Can you please explain what energy centers, or chakras, are and how they can help
us heal and evolve spiritually? Also, I've heard that there are only seven chakras.
Can you explain what the eighth and ninth chakras are?

Chakra is a term derived from Sanskrit that means "wheel." The word "chakra" is often used to describe the various spinning wheels of energy oscillating at different frequencies around the body. Seven of the major chakras are located within a subtle body called the "etheric body."

Chakras contain emotional, mental, energetic, ancestral, cellular, and spiritual information. They are part of our energetic anatomy and can provide vital information about potential physical problems before they occur. The energy flow that moves in and out of the chakras interacts with various energy bodies surrounding our physical body. These energy centers are also influenced by our interactions with our environment, other people, and Universal Intelligence.

In this chapter, you will learn that by working on each energy center, you can improve your health, relationships, abundance, and self-esteem, as well as let go of fear, guilt, and shame. You can also develop your intuition, open your heart, communicate more effectively, deepen your connection with the Divine, experience peace, and draw miracles into your life.

Tuning In

When we are unwell or out of balance, our chakras slow down and store dense energy. A person skilled in sensing subtle energy can immediately see the mental, emotional, and physical problems that someone is experiencing by tuning in to their chakras.

In Eastern cultures, chakra healing has been used for thousands of years to heal physical, emotional, and energetic disturbances.

My ability to tune in to subtle energy systems has given me a direct experience of how chakras look and feel, and the information they contain. I've also asked children, who are skilled at scanning the body, to tune in to their own and others' chakras and describe what they saw. Even though they didn't know much about the chakra system, they conveyed many of the same feelings, colors, and insights that I had received. Thus, I feel confident in sharing my discoveries with you.

Anyone Can Learn How to Work with Chakras

What is important to understand is that anyone who is open and willing to learn can improve their well-being by working with their chakras. This practice is not only for people with special abilities. Although many individuals might be skeptical about their capacity to tune in to their own or someone else's chakras, in my years of teaching, I have rarely met people who cannot receive information from the energy centers when given the correct guidance.

While I have taught people who have a more natural ability than others, everyone who has persevered has been able to tune in to their own and other people's energy systems, receive messages, and heal.

Chakra Clearing Processes

Following each description of a chakra, there is a simple chakra clearing process that you can either do separately for each chakra or one after the other. You may also like to hold a crystal related to each chakra and meditate on it for a few minutes, being open to any wisdom or insights that may occur to you; or you may want to place the crystal on the part of your body related to the chakra. You can sit, lie, or even stand while doing the chakra clearing processes. The most important thing is to be comfortable and to make time for your self-healing.

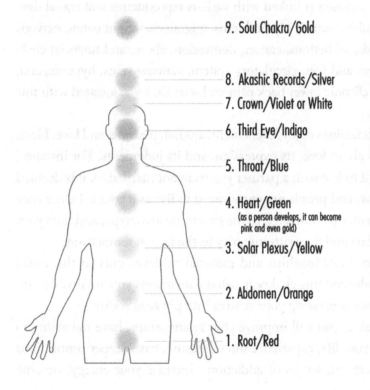

9. Soul Chakra/Gold

8. Akashic Records/Silver

7. Crown/Violet or White

6. Third Eye/Indigo

5. Throat/Blue

4. Heart/Green
(as a person develops, it can become
pink and even gold)

3. Solar Plexus/Yellow

2. Abdomen/Orange

1. Root/Red

In addition, I have recorded a more in-depth healing audio program, called "Nine Chakras," that you can purchase from InnaSegal.com and use in conjunction with the descriptions and processes below.

First Chakra—Root

The first chakra, also known as the base or root chakra, is located around the lower hips and genital area. The dominant color of the first chakra is red.

This chakra is responsible for the fight-or-flight response, and holds many of our thoughts, feelings, programs, and imprints from our family and other groups we associate with. Some of our deepest and earliest patterns are stored here, as well as our issues surrounding survival, sexuality, safety, and security. This chakra contains feelings of superiority and inferiority, loyalty, family beliefs, superstitions, traditions, rituals, as well as the power we have in our community, or the lack thereof.

The root chakra contains physical and emotional trauma—feelings of fear, rage, and terror. Much of people's life force energy is kept in this chakra and can either be channeled into fear and stress or passion and love. It is a very important chakra to work with in terms of self-healing, as it can give us the courage, the conviction, and the energy required to heal.

On the physical level, this chakra is linked with various reproductive and sexual dysfunctions and diseases, compulsive eating, hip problems, migraines, weight issues, nervous system disorders, hemorrhoids, addictions, cancer, depression, abuse, and financial challenges. Problems with the legs and feet, circulatory system, varicose veins, hypertension, and inflammation, as well as chronic lower back pain and sciatica, are associated with this energy center.

The root chakra also holds feelings of joy, excitement, arousal, pleasure, and love. Here, we often carry societal ideals about love, its expression, and its judgments. For instance, although it was once shameful to live with a partner you were not married to, it is deemed normal in many societies now, and people are encouraged to live as a couple before they plunge into marriage. This center is connected to the prostitute archetype, and tests your willingness to follow your heart and live with integrity in the face of temptation.

Often, the success of your relationships and material achievements in the world depends on how clear and balanced this chakra is, what convictions you are invested in, and how confident you are in manifesting your desires into physical reality.

By clearing your root chakra, you will improve your relationships, have the ability to attract more abundance into your life, experience more pleasure, have deeper connections with others, raise your self-esteem, let go of addictions, increase your energy, become more grounded, and heal.

Process for Clearing Your Root Chakra

Crystal to work with—Garnet

Close your eyes. Stand up. Take a lingering deep breath, hold it for a count of seven, and slowly exhale. Repeat this breathing exercise four to six times.

Rub your hands together vigorously for about a minute. Place your palms next to each other without touching. You will most likely feel a tingling sensation. Visualize holding a large red ball of energy between your hands. Focus on this ball of energy and allow it to intensify. Play with this color for about thirty seconds, exploring how far you can extend its energy by widening the distance between your hands.

Place your hands in front of your first chakra, which is located around the lower hips and genital area, without touching your body. Take deep, slow breaths, inhaling this red light. Visualize the red light moving through your root chakra, clearing any density and rejuvenating your chakra.

Say: "Divine Healing Intelligence, please assist me in gently releasing any deep feelings of fear, shame, insecurity, shock, or any other painful patterns stored in my root chakra. Help me improve my current relationships, attract abundance, and increase my self-esteem, and allow me to experience deep joy and satisfaction in every area of my life. Thank you."

Repeat the word "CLEAR" several times with the intention of releasing any negativity and amplifying any positive aspects.

Relax your hands. Sit down. Visualize or think about what it would be like if you were treated exactly the way you would love by the people you care about. Imagine feeling confident and doing things that make you happy. Spend a few minutes focusing on what makes you happy in your life.

Place both hands in front of your pubic bone. Your middle fingers should touch while the other fingers point toward each other, almost touching. As you take a deep breath, focus on your lower abdomen and expand it. When you exhale, contract your stomach muscles as well as the muscles of your perineum. Do this several times. As you breathe, focus on grounding yourself by concentrating your attention on your feet. Stay in this position as long as you feel comfortable.

Second Chakra—Sacral
The second chakra, also known as the sacral chakra, is located just beneath the navel. It is our creative and emotional center. The dominant color of the second chakra is orange.

In the sacral chakra, we store feelings of guilt, fear, blame, control, and anger. It also carries money and sexual issues, and feelings of powerlessness and victimhood.

Here, we yearn to have loving, fulfilling, passionate, and nourishing relationships. We also desire to be attractive, appealing, and fascinating. This is the center where we most fear losing control, being humiliated, and shamed.

On the physical level, the sacral chakra is linked to intestinal problems, appendix disorders, indigestion, gout, hernias, irritable bowel, kidney problems, hypertension, inflammation, psoriasis, chronic lower back pain, childhood issues, fertility issues, and women's issues, such as PMS, candida, ovarian disorders, uterine problems, pelvic pain, frigidity, ovarian cancers, rigidity, frozen shoulders, and acne. Male issues such as impotence, baldness, male fertility, and prostate problems are also stored here.

While the root chakra contains our ancestral fears and beliefs, the sacral influences our capacity to handle money, success, sexual energies, and the ability to influence others. Some of the above issues are shared within both energy centers.

The sacral chakra helps us to interpret others' feelings, make judgments about our own feelings and creativity, and either lose or increase our life force energy. It is connected to the inner-child archetype and our feelings around survival. Instinctually, we are constantly using this center to check whether we and our loved ones are emotionally, physically, and financially secure and protected. Through this chakra, we can attempt to manipulate and control others in order to get what we want.

Here, we also store our cravings and addictions. We lose power by giving it to an authority outside of ourselves, whether it is a romantic partner, drugs, food, alcohol, family members, or work colleagues. And we fear the loss of love, money, health, beauty, power, and life.

Additionally, the sacral chakra is a storehouse of violation; jealousy; power games; and emotional, mental, and physical abuse. Our deepest vulnerabilities lie here, including the fear that there is something acutely wrong with us. We dread being alone, isolated, and rejected, thus we blame and project our guilt onto others. We also wear masks in order to conceal our shadow aspects and display virtuousness—to gain love and approval so that we feel better about ourselves. We yearn to feel forever youthful, useful, and attractive. Much of the billion-dollar beauty, antiaging, weight-loss, fitness, and dating industries are built upon the desires and insecurities we carry in this chakra.

By working on and clearing the sacral chakra, you will be able to let go of fear, sorrow, worry, guilt, anger, shame, self-punishment, and being a victim or a pleaser. You will develop your inner power, perseverance, and resilience; experience an increase in energy; have deeper, more intimate sensual relationships; increase your confidence; open up to feelings of happiness; and embrace life. You will also create healthy relationships with others, enhance your self-worth, and express yourself more creatively.

Process for Clearing Your Sacral Chakra

Crystal to work with—Carnelian

Rub your hands together vigorously for about sixty seconds. Place your palms next to each other without touching. You will most likely feel a tingling sensation. Visualize holding a large orange ball of energy between your hands. Focus on this ball of energy and allow it to intensify. Play with this color for about thirty seconds, exploring how far you can extend its energy by widening the distance between your hands.

Place your hands in front of your navel without actually touching your body. Take slow, deep breaths and inhale this orange light. Visualize how the orange light moves through your chakra and begins to clear and dissolve any density, rejuvenating your sacral chakra.

Say: "Divine Healing Intelligence, please assist me to gently release any feelings of guilt, fear, sorrow, worry, blame, powerlessness, anger, and any other painful patterns that are stored in my sacral chakra. Strengthen my inner power, resilience, creative abilities, and belief in myself. Allow me to become friends with my feelings and to listen to my inner guidance. Thank you."

Repeat the word "CLEAR" several times with the intention of releasing any negativity and amplifying any positive aspects.

Relax your hands and give yourself permission to be imaginative. If you could be free to express your creativity in any way you desire, what would you do? What can you do this week that is creative and will make your life more interesting and productive? If you are trying to find a solution to a challenging situation, allow a creative idea to float into your mind.

Interlace the fingers of both your hands and place them just beneath your navel. Take long, slow, lingering breaths and focus on finding the perfect avenues to express your creative abilities. Stay in this position as long as you feel comfortable.

Third Chakra—Solar Plexus

The third chakra, also known as the solar plexus chakra, is located below the sternum in the area of the diaphragm, and is known as our personal power center. The dominant color of the third chakra is yellow.

This chakra stores our beliefs, judgments, feelings, fears, hopes, and dreams. The combination of our experiences, sensitivities, and opinions affects how we view ourselves, the people around us, and the opportunities we attract.

As many of our interactions with others are experienced through our solar plexus chakra, we need to develop self-confidence, self-respect, and self-understanding. People decide how to treat us by subconsciously tuning in to our personal power center and sensing how we feel about ourselves. The more our beliefs, emotions, and actions are aligned, the more other people hold us in high regard. However, if we keep nourishing our fears and insecurities, they are more likely to exploit and mistreat us.

We use our solar plexus chakra to become aware of other people's motives. Depending on whether we feel threatened or safe, the rest of our centers either contract or open.

Our inner critic is expressed through this chakra. If given too much power, it can be detrimental to our lives and creative pursuits, with its constant put downs and procrastination on important decisions.

On the physical level, this chakra is linked to stomach problems, diabetes, arthritis, adrenal exhaustion, metabolic disorders, weight issues, anorexia, bulimia, obesity, indigestion, liver problems, hepatitis, spleen disorders, and gallbladder problems.

The solar plexus chakra helps us to develop a healthy relationship with ourselves and take positive action toward our goals. It is connected to the victim archetype, which either makes us lose our power or helps us become victorious and successful.

Our integrity (or lack of it) is linked to this center. The question of integrity can be challenging, depending on our point of view, where we grew up, and what we value. Life often tests our feelings of righteousness by placing us in situations similar to those of the ones we have judged. As there is often no black and white in life, the potential here is to be soft and forgiving with ourselves and others. This chakra gives us an opportunity to examine how we lose and gain energy, and adjust our choices accordingly.

By working with this chakra, you can increase your self-esteem, enhance your inner power, and learn to use your intuition. This is the center where you develop trust and take responsibility for your actions. When clear, it allows you to experience independence and to make optimal decisions. You also become conscious of where, how, and with whom you need to draw boundaries and clarify how you believe you should be treated.

Process for Clearing Your Solar Plexus Chakra

Crystal to work with—Citrine

Rub your hands together vigorously for about sixty seconds. Place your palms next to each other without touching. You will most likely feel a tingling sensation. Visualize holding a large yellow ball of energy between your hands. Focus on this ball of energy and allow it to intensify. Play with this color for about thirty seconds, exploring how far you can extend its energy by widening the distance between your hands.

Place your hands in front of your solar plexus without touching your body. Take deep, slow breaths, and inhale this yellow light.

Visualize the yellow light moving through your chakra and beginning to clear and dissolve any density, rejuvenating your solar plexus chakra.

Say: "Divine Healing Intelligence, please assist me to gently release any judgments, low self-esteem, resentment, victimhood, confusion, power issues, control issues, and any other painful patterns that are stored in my solar plexus chakra. Increase my intuitive abilities and assist me to trust in the Divine Intelligence that is guiding my life. Help me become more independent, empowered, clear, and successful. Thank you."

Repeat the word "CLEAR" several times with the intention of releasing any negativity and amplifying any positive aspects.

Relax your hands and focus on what it would be like—how it would feel—to make empowering decisions and behave in a powerful way for the highest good of all. Become aware of how you can begin to listen to your intuition and to trust it. Ask your Higher Self to increase your intuition so that you can hear it clearly. Give yourself permission to act on your intuition daily.

Place the palms of your hands together, fingers spread apart, and lift them to the level of your solar plexus. This is a position of power and decisiveness. As you slowly inhale, press your fingers together and focus on your strength and commitment to succeed. As you exhale, relax your fingers and focus on letting go of any tension and resistance to success. Do this for two to three minutes.

Fourth Chakra—Heart

The fourth chakra, also known as the heart chakra, is located around your chest and is seen as the love and relationship center. The dominant color of the fourth chakra is green.

The heart chakra is the center of love, openness, and compassion; our soul communicates with us through our heart and our passion for life. The more we develop our connection with the heart chakra, the more fulfilling, sweet, prosperous, joyful, enriched, and warm our lives will be.

Our ability to forgive, heal, evolve, and transform are the keys to opening the heart chakra. This chakra is strongly linked to the root chakra and our capacity to manifest from a place of passion, love, and truth. As we evolve, we increase our ability to release our judgments and to perceive events and experiences from our heart and soul. Our relationships also begin to transform from those based on jealousy and ownership to soulful, unconditional connections not bound by time and space. We start to embrace the Divine Wisdom of the higher chakras.

On the physical level, this chakra is linked to heart problems, circulatory disease, blood clotting, heart attack, blood pressure problems, asthma, bronchitis, pneumonia, lung and breast cancer, allergies, shoulder and arm problems, insomnia, immune system disorders, and lymphoma.

This chakra holds feelings of love, hate, loneliness, resentment, bitterness, grief, and anger. This is also where we feel compassion, forgiveness, hope, and trust. It is connected to the saboteur archetype, which can either guard our hearts and sabotage nourishing relationships or lead us to heart-opening, loving experiences while protecting us from potentially abusive people.

Clearing the heart chakra improves your relationships, attracts love into your life, and helps you discover your purpose. When you are connected with your heart center, it guides you to the most powerful and loving experiences. If you are in a relationship, it greatly enhances it and opens the lines of communication. It also allows fun, joy, laughter, and love to come into your life. This is a center of inspired creativity and communion with the Divine; the heart can uplift and transform a human life. Caring touch, loving hugs, and true sharing heal the heart. By opening your heart chakra, you have the capacity to live your life from a consciousness of unconditional love, which deeply empowers others.

Process for Clearing Your Heart Chakra

Crystal to work with—Emerald

Rub your hands together vigorously for about a minute. Place your palms next to each other without touching. You will most likely feel a tingling sensation. Visualize holding a large green ball of energy between your hands. Focus on this ball of energy and allow it to intensify. Play with this color for about thirty seconds, exploring how far you can extend its energy by widening the distance between your hands.

Place your hands in front of your heart without touching your body. Take deep slow breaths, and inhale this green light.

Visualize the green light moving through your chakra, clearing and dissolving any density, and rejuvenating your heart chakra.

Say: "Divine Healing Intelligence, please assist me to gently release any feelings of loneliness, anger, resentment, grief, loss, heartache, depression, and any other painful patterns that are stored in my heart chakra. Awaken my passion, enthusiasm, and zest for life. Allow me to attract and experience the deepest, most loving, fulfilling, compassionate relationships. Thank you."

Repeat the word "CLEAR" several times with the intention of releasing any negativity and amplifying any positive aspects.

Relax your hands and focus on how joyful it would be to have open, loving, deep connections to others. If you already feel this, allow your heart to open and expand as you focus on the people you love. Feel the energy of love as it heals and re-energizes you. If you do not feel connected to your heart or do not have loving relationships, focus on allowing your heart to open and attract the relationships you would love to experience.

Place your hands on your heart and gently massage it in a circular motion. Give thanks to your heart for keeping you alive. Focus on all the things you are deeply grateful for. In your mind's eye, allow your heart to grow, expand, and fill with wisdom. Imagine that this wisdom moves from your heart into your mind, connecting these two aspects of yourself through a gold string of light. What would it be like if you could embrace the wisdom of your heart and the intelligence of your mind to make important decisions in your life?

Fifth Chakra—Throat

The fifth chakra, also known as the throat chakra, is located in the front of your throat, and is seen as the communication center. The dominant color of the fifth chakra is blue.

The throat chakra is the area that helps us make important decisions, become accountable for our behavior, receive guidance, and share our wisdom. We manifest things into physical reality using this chakra, by having a clear intention, expressing ourselves, and taking action. This is also where we hold responsibilities, judgments, and criticisms about ourselves and others.

This center deals with self-expression. It allows us to be creative, make powerful choices, and ask for what we want. It gives us the opportunity to say yes or no. The throat chakra helps us to develop our confidence and voice. Here, we explore our influence, and the ability to keep our word and to support others. Breaking our word or commitment can create emotional and energetic scars in ourselves and others—scars that may remain for many years and lead to illness.

Vows taken at the level of the fifth chakra have the power to dominate our lives: vows to change, give up smoking, be of service, or take care of ourselves. They can also be taken when we desire higher help to be saved from something difficult or to gain a miracle. On the other hand, if we live our lives from a space of fear, we can carry vows to live in poverty, suffer in silence, struggle, put up with abuse, or be a slave to others. In religious orders, people can take vows to be of service to others or in order to raise their own consciousness.

Through constant misunderstandings of one another and a lack of clear communication, we lose our soul fragments and end up feeling frustrated, limited, and disempowered. Many spiritual and religious traditions, particularly shamanism, teach the practice of recovering our soul fragments in order to regain the full power of our soul wisdom, clear and regenerate our bodies, raise our life force energy, and retrieve our past gifts and abilities. By retrieving our soul fragments, we can learn to communicate in a clear and aware manner, taking the circumstance, time, and people involved into consideration, and speaking in a manner they can receive.

On the physical level, this chakra is linked to throat and mouth problems, such as a chronic sore throat, ulcers, gum problems, tooth decay, swollen glands, and laryngitis, as well as high blood pressure, inflammation, fever, infection, headache, neck problems, goiter, hyperthyroidism, thyroid disorder, depression, iodine deficiency, hypothalamic dysfunction, and insomnia.

Many people store feelings of helplessness and victimization here, or they simply hold everything in and don't communicate. This is also a center where people can feel a compulsive need to control themselves, people they care about, their finances, or other external events.

As most people hold a lot of fear in their throat chakra, it can be easy to allow emotional manipulation, to embrace old superstitions, and to participate in outdated customs. This energy center also gives us an opportunity for liberation and freedom of expression.

By clearing the throat chakra, you improve your communication and manifestation abilities, allowing you to be more confident, creative, empowered, and clear in the choices you make. The challenge here is to connect the wisdom of your mind with the love of your heart and share this with others. You have an opportunity to listen to and apply others' insights as long as these resonate with your inner self. Working with the throat chakra also intensifies your capacity to connect to your soul wisdom and to attract the opportunities necessary to express your soul purpose.

Process for Clearing Your Throat Chakra

Crystal to work with—Turquoise

Rub your hands together vigorously for about a minute. Place your palms next to each other without touching. You will most likely feel a tingling sensation. Visualize holding a large blue ball of energy between your hands. Focus on this ball of energy and allow it to intensify. Play with this color for about thirty seconds, exploring how far you can extend its energy by widening the distance between your hands.

Position your hands in front of your throat without touching your body. Take deep, slow breaths, and inhale this blue light.

Visualize the blue light moving through your chakra, clearing and dissolving any density and rejuvenating your throat chakra.

Say: "Divine Healing Intelligence, please assist me to gently release any self-criticism, fear, inability to express myself, low self-worth, guilt, suppression, and any other painful patterns that are stored in my throat chakra. Help me to become more honest with myself and others about my desires and intentions. Give me confidence to clearly express myself and skillfully communicate with others. Allow my greatest desires to flow into my life, at perfect moments and in perfect ways. Thank you."

Repeat the word "CLEAR" several times with the intention of releasing any negativity and amplifying any positive aspects.

Relax your hands. Imagine talking to someone in your life to whom you need to express something important that you have been avoiding. Imagine that this person is listening intently to what you are saying and understands your point of view. When you feel ready, if it is possible, express it to him or her in real life. Remember, it is important that you articulate how you feel with compassion. When you communicate clearly and live honestly, you become healthier, more joyful, and fulfilled.

Lift your arms to the level of your throat. Grasp your fingers. (Your right palm should face outward and your left palm toward you.) Pull your hands as if you are trying to pull them apart. Make sure you keep your shoulders down. Inhale deeply and hum either *haaaaa* or *ommmmm* on your out breath. This posture allows you to strengthen and empower your voice.

Sixth Chakra—Third Eye

The sixth chakra is also known as the third eye chakra. It is located in the middle of the forehead and is seen as the center of intuition, inspiration, and wisdom. The dominant color of the sixth chakra is indigo.

This chakra allows us to tune in to our inner world, and connect to our guidance, to receive messages, interpret those messages, and to decide how to act on these messages. This center helps us connect to our mental body and develop a focused, clear, and disciplined mind, bringing our dreams and visions into reality. We constantly use this chakra to evaluate whether our goals are realistic, doable, and financially viable.

Many of our hormonal and endocrine operations are influenced by the third eye chakra, which has a profound effect on our emotions and behaviors.

On the physical level, this chakra is linked to brain tumors, strokes, neurological problems, glandular or endocrine issues, hormonal imbalances, issues with eyesight (like blindness), deafness, sinus problems, spinal difficulties, learning disabilities, seizures, and headaches.

Through this center, we create our self-image and connect to our higher wisdom.

We also discover our truth—what really resonates with us and what doesn't—develop our mental and spiritual intelligence, and open ourselves up to new ideas. Our imagination and what we believe is possible reside here. We can utilize the power of the third eye chakra by combining our visualization skills with positive intention and confident action. If we are unwell, this chakra can assist us in healing by helping us to connect to our Divine Energy, tune in to our bodies, release any hurtful experiences we still carry, and change our cellular memories by adjusting how we interpreted an experience.

By clearing this chakra, you open your clairvoyant ability and receive important information from the past, present, and future. You also improve your vision and hearing, feel more balanced, increase your capacity for learning, and develop your wisdom and intuition. By connecting to this chakra, you can give valuable insights to others and help them regain their faith and confidence. You can access the big picture in various situations and detach from negativity, threat, and fear, focusing your attention on faith, inner exploration, and higher powers.

The intention of this center is to help you become spiritually, mentally, emotionally, and physically congruent; live in the present; and appreciate your life. If you work on evolving your consciousness, then the objective is to let go of all your mental or emotional preferences and live your life in harmony with the Divine Will. Success at the level of this chakra means discovering the highest truth, working on any difficulties that arise, and constantly looking for the blessings in every situation you encounter.

Process for Clearing Your Third Eye Chakra

Crystal to work with—Amethyst

Rub your hands together vigorously for about a minute. Place your palms next to each other without touching. You will most likely feel a tingling sensation. Visualize holding a large indigo ball of energy between your hands. Focus on this ball of energy and allow it to intensify. Play with this color for about thirty seconds, exploring how far you can extend its energy by widening the distance between your hands.

Place your hands in front of your third eye without touching your body. Take deep slow breaths and inhale this indigo light.

Visualize the indigo light moving through your chakra, clearing and dissolving any density, and rejuvenating your third eye chakra.

Say: "Divine Healing Intelligence, please help me gently release any internal confusion, imbalance, lack of direction, frustration, limitation, fear, stress, resistance, and any other painful patterns that are stored in my third eye chakra. Help me to open my third eye and increase my intuitive ability. Inspire me to listen to my intuition and follow my Divine Guidance and inspiration. Allow me to live my life from a truthful, balanced, joyful, spiritual perspective. Thank you."

Repeat the word "CLEAR" several times with the intention of releasing any negativity and amplifying any positive aspects.

Rub your third eye with your middle finger for about a minute in a circular motion. Concentrate on activating your intuition and having clarity in an area of your life where you are currently experiencing confusion. Do this until you feel open and receptive to intuitive guidance.

Seventh Chakra—Crown

The seventh chakra, also known as the crown chakra, is located around the top of the head and is seen as the center for higher intelligence. The dominant colors of the seventh chakra are white or violet.

This chakra is related to the area at the top of the head, the brain, the pineal gland, and the entire nervous system. It is our connection to Divinity, spirituality, and synchronicity. Through this center, we can develop miracle mindedness, connect to our higher purpose, and discover our unity with all life.

With meditation, prayer, and the surrender of our limitations and fears, we can transcend the illusionary and egoic mind and enter the infinite field of consciousness. We can experience miracle healings, transcendental states of consciousness, and Divine Inspiration.

The crown chakra absorbs Divine Energy, which nourishes all the systems, organs, and centers of the body. The clearer this chakra, the more life force energy we can enjoy.

This center is associated with energetic disorders, chronic exhaustion, immune system disorders, major depression, cancers, sexual dysfunction, hypertension, muscular system disorders, bone and skeletal problems, blood problems, fibromyalgia, dizziness, Parkinson's disease, paralysis, epilepsy, multiple personality disorders, multiple sclerosis, schizophrenia, and dementia.

The crown chakra gives us the ability to see the larger aspects of life. We develop our capacity for devotion, spiritual healing, and evolution here. This is also where we can experience the dark night of the soul, where we may feel alone, abandoned, and disconnected from all that is soulful, loving, and Divine. This often occurs when someone endures an emotional crisis or a physical trauma; witnesses or participates in a natural disaster or war; discovers that they have an incurable illness; or suffers a loss of a loved one, either through death, heartbreak, or a dispute.

The dark night experience can also arise when a person moves through the stages required to fully surrender to Divinity. This may arouse feelings of deep isolation, depression, fear, loneliness, and nothingness, as well as bliss, oneness, peace, all-encompassing understanding, and illumination. Our ability to keep the faith and exercise our courage, even in the most difficult situations, matures in this chakra.

Because it is connected to higher realities, the seventh chakra constantly evaluates whether our choices are for our highest good and serve our Divine potential. Many of the greatest visions and inventions were accessed through the crown chakra. Meditation and self-healing are excellent ways to transcend ordinary human limitations into extraordinary possibilities. The information we are able to access in this chakra is mystical, nonlinear, and visionary.

Clearing this chakra will allow you to experience a profound connection to the Divine, help you to follow your life purpose, give you a deeper ability to understand others, have greater compassion, and experience oneness. When your crown chakra is clear, you may experience higher states of consciousness, access your healing ability, and receive messages from the Divine. You will also feel more balanced, stronger, healthier, and more alive.

Process for Clearing Your Crown Chakra

Crystal to work with—Clear Quartz

Rub your hands together vigorously for about a minute. Place your palms next to each other without touching. You will most likely feel a tingling sensation. Visualize holding a large white ball of energy between your hands. Focus on this ball of energy and allow it to intensify. Play with this color for about thirty seconds, exploring how far you can extend its energy by widening the distance between your hands.

Place your hands above your head without touching your body. Take slow, deep breaths and inhale this white light.

Visualize the white light moving through your chakra, beginning to clear and dissolving any density in your crown chakra, and rejuvenating it.

Say: "Divine Healing Intelligence, please help me to release any stress, exhaustion, disconnection from my Divinity, fear, worry, confusion, depression, loss of direction, and any other painful patterns that are stored in my crown chakra. Help me to bolster my immune system and cleanse my nervous system. Give me access to higher understanding and the ability to see a bigger picture. Deepen my connection with the Divine and allow me to experience higher states of consciousness. Awaken my love, compassion, and kindness toward myself and others. Thank you."

Repeat the word "CLEAR" several times with the intention of releasing any negativity and amplifying any positive aspects.

Interlace your fingers without touching your palms and place your hands just above your head, with the thumbs just touching your hair. Extend your thumbs away from your index fingers and feel the pulsing vibration move through your thumbs. Hold for one to two minutes while focusing on energizing your crown chakra. Take slow, deep breaths and focus on breathing in purity, clarity, and ease. Take a minute to meditate on your connection with the Divinity of life. Then lower your hands in front of your heart, with your thumbs extended toward your heart and the rest of the fingers still interlaced. Meditate for one or two minutes about all you are grateful for in your life.

Eighth Chakra—Akashic Records

This chakra, also known as the Akashic Records chakra, is located about four centimeters (about one and a half inches) above the head. This is where the Akashic Records, the cosmic "books" that contain records of all we have ever experienced (saw, felt, said, thought, or done in the past, present, and future), are kept.

Many believe the Akashic Records are similar to the idea of collective consciousness. We can gain access about our past and other lifetimes through this chakra. The Akashic Records chakra has information about our karma, the issues we have come to deal with, and the lessons we have come to learn. We can also gain understanding of many of our patterns through this chakra, making it an invaluable resource for healing chronic physical pain, past traumas, and karmic relationships.

On the physical level, an eighth chakra imbalance makes us feel dizzy and dissociated, affects our immune system; and causes metabolic problems, weight issues, fatigue, tremors, throat and thyroid problems, eye issues, ear problems, and depression. Disease and unresolved emotional issues can also be carried over from previous lifetimes—especially those related to abandonment, rejection, and lack of self-worth.

This is the center that regulates our destiny. Here, we have the power to make new choices, and to release the vows and soul agreements that no longer serve us, while honoring those that do. We can also access our talents, past ability, and the confidence to move toward our soul purpose.

We have the opportunity to connect to our soul mates and discover unconditional love, Divine devotion, and oneness through this chakra. Our soul mates can help us grow, evolve, release limitations and judgments, and experience higher states of consciousness. They can also help us remember, understand, and heal our past lives and karmic patterns. This is an area from which it is important to clear or possibly dissolve energy cords with people with whom we have had difficult or abusive relationships.

By clearing this chakra, you can release negative and limiting energy passed down to you by your ancestors, improve your relationships, release chronic problems, and gain access to important information about your past and future. By releasing hurt and pain from your past, you can experience more peace and clarity in the present. You can also open your heart to the most extraordinary connections, higher consciousness, and love.

Grounding yourself is extremely important after working with this chakra, as you don't want to get lost in fantasies of what has happened or what you wish to occur.

Process for Clearing Your Akashic Records Chakra

Crystal to work with—Snowflake Obsidian

Rub your hands together vigorously for about a minute. Place your palms next to each other without touching. You will most likely feel a tingling sensation. Visualize holding a large silver ball of energy between your hands. Focus on this ball of energy and allow it to intensify. Play with this color for about thirty seconds, exploring how far you can extend its energy by widening the distance between your hands.

Place your hands (palms down) about four centimeters (one and a half inches) above your head without touching your body. Take slow, deep breaths; inhale this silver light.

Visualize the silver light moving through your chakra, beginning to clear and dissolving any density, and rejuvenating your Akashic Records chakra. Imagine silver light moving through all your chakras like a light rain.

Say: "Divine Healing Intelligence, help me release any negative chronic patterns, heaviness, or physical challenges that I no longer need. Show me how to grow and expand through ease, joy, and enthusiasm. Help me understand my soul's purpose and give me the tools to fulfill it. Lead me toward becoming a powerful, responsible cocreator of my life. Bring to me my soul mates and people who can help me open my heart, understand my soul, and evolve. Thank you."

Repeat the word "CLEAR" several times with the intention of releasing any negativity and amplifying any positive aspects.

Meditate on the Akashic Records chakra. Ask to receive any images or messages about the past, present, or future that can assist you in experiencing more meaning in your life now or in the near future. Give yourself permission to embrace and use any particular talent or ability you are trying to develop. If you can't think of any talents you may have, ask to know yourself deeper.

Visualize that you have a blank piece of paper in front of you. In your imagination, write or draw anything that you would like to experience. Always write or intend that things happen with ease and grace for the highest good of all. Ask that you either receive what you asked for or something better. When you have done that, imagine putting this paper into an old book that represents your Akashic Records. Be open to having your intentions manifest.

Ninth Chakra—Soul Chakra

This chakra, also known as the soul chakra, is located approximately an arm's length above the head. The soul chakra reveals important truths about our health and lifestyle through images, symbols, numbers, archetypes, metaphors, colors, shapes, feelings, codes, sounds, vibrations, sacred geometry, and dreams.

The soul chakra contains inspiration for our soul and life purpose, the soul agreements we have made, and the steps we need to take to fulfill our objectives.

Often, when healers, medical intuitives, or psychotherapists connect to this chakra, they are shown metaphoric images of what is happening in a person's life. These images can tell a full story of a person's current physical and emotional state through one or more clear pictures, demonstrating whether they are on the right track or have gone off their soul path and need to readjust their direction. Often, health practitioners tune in to this chakra without being consciously aware that this is where they receive their most valuable information.

On the physical level, we can experience fatigue when our soul chakra is imbalanced, as we may have lost many of our soul fragments or possibly did not bring enough of our soul energy into the physical experience.

By exploring the soul chakra, we can understand what roles our archetypal companions play in our lives. In other words, who is driving our symbolic bus—the prostitute, inner child, victim, saboteur, mystic, healer, slave, judge, or another archetype? It gives us profound insights into our shadow and light aspects.

Through this chakra, we begin to learn more about our soul, its intentions, and the role we perform in the spirit world when we are between physical lives—as well as our level of evolution. We also have an opportunity to understand our soul's choices, including why we chose our time and place of birth, body, parents, life experiences and challenges, financial conditions, and so forth. This chakra contains the soul programs regarding our physical, emotional, mental, and spiritual experiences.

By clearing and regenerating your soul chakra, which transmits information from one reality into another, you can ensure that you learn and assimilate the appropriate lessons and experiences you have come to understand; you can make new and empowering choices that uplift you and humanity at large. Here, you become aware that there is truly only one of us, so anything that affects you influences others, and vice versa. The more you connect to this chakra, the more you will feel like being of service to others, and making a difference from your heart and soul.

By continually working with the soul chakra, you have ready access to the knowledge of your soul destiny and can receive inspiration about the steps you need to take to fulfill your life purpose.

Your guides and angelic helpers often make their presence known to you during meditations or visions when you are in tune with this chakra.

When you explore your soul chakra and higher levels of consciousness, you move out of linear reality and draw synchronicities, miracles, and mystical experiences into your life.

Process for Clearing Your Soul Chakra

Crystal to work with—Gold with Quartz

Rub your hands together vigorously for about a minute. Place your palms next to each other without touching. You will most likely feel a tingling sensation. Visualize holding a gold ball of energy between your hands. Focus on this ball of energy and allow it to intensify. Play with this color for about thirty seconds, exploring how far you can extend its energy by widening the distance between your hands.

Raise your hands above your head at arm's length. Take slow, deep breaths and inhale this gold light.

Visualize the gold light moving through your chakra, beginning to clear and dissolve any density, and rejuvenating your soul chakra. Visualize the gold light moving through all your chakras like a light rain.

Say: "Divine Healing Intelligence, please help me release any negative, limiting, and disempowering beliefs that I may carry about who I am and my self-worth. Help me reconnect to my Divinity and soulfulness. Assist me in hearing my spiritual guides and helpers, and let me learn any lessons I am here to discover. Show me that my challenges are really blessings in disguise, and help me find peace. Thank you."

Repeat the word "CLEAR" several times with the intention of releasing any negativity and amplifying any positive aspects.

Relax your arms and close your eyes. Take slow, deep breaths, and allow yourself to meditate and slow down. Remind yourself that you are not alone, and ask your spiritual helpers to assist you to resolve whatever challenge you are facing. Some people feel or see their helpers easily; others may need more time to open up and trust. Remember, your spiritual helpers love you unconditionally and have infinite patience; their intention is only to help and support you. Keep strengthening your connection with them and be open to receiving the answers you are looking for, even if these arrive in a different package than what you had expected.

Helping Each Other to Heal

By understanding and clearing your chakras, you not only work with energy that can help you heal your body but you also simultaneously transform how you live your life.

Deepak Chopra, in his book *Reinventing the Body, Resurrecting the Soul*, states, "The biggest excitement centers on finding new genes, matching them with specific disease, then trying to manipulate or splice them before harm is done to the body. Yet the start should have been energy, because germs and genes, like any object, are reducible to energy, and therefore, all harm caused to the body is traceable to this fundamental force."[4]

I am always really impressed at the end of each Visionary Intuitive Healing® workshop I teach, when I see people tuning in to each other's chakras and accessing important and often astonishingly accurate information about the state of each other's physical, mental, and emotional well-being.

It is even more thrilling to see people healing each other's longstanding physical, emotional, and mental patterns and pain by gently working with the chakra system. The following is a healing experience shared by Adam, who attended several of my Visionary Intuitive Healing® workshops. Adam had never done any type of healing work before coming to my seminars. It is impressive to note that Adam was able to see images that he could interpret and share with Monica, and help her to not only heal her physical pain and release a lot of emotional stagnation, but to also free her mother, who had passed over.

Adam's Story: Tuning in to Help Monica Heal

I am a fashion designer, and I use Visionary Intuitive Healing® every day for my personal well-being and balance. I also do healings for family or friends who specifically ask for help. Recently, a close friend asked me if I would see Monica, her cousin, who was having a very difficult time.

When I saw Monica, she was visibly in a lot of pain; her neck and shoulders were very sore. She had been living on painkillers for months, but they no longer helped. And although an osteopath had managed to alleviate the pain temporarily, it returned a few days later. She was also plagued by stomach cramps and digestive problems, which often prevented her from eating and sleeping.

When I tuned in to her throat chakra, I saw a thick harness made of dense black bands attached to her neck with a thick chain that was pulled tight. All her energy was being pulled backwards, leaving her feeling as if she was about to keel over.

When I tried to ease the tension on the chain, I saw that it was held by an elderly lady, and I clearly heard the word "mother." Three smaller chains were attached from the throat chakra to the second chakra in the stomach area, which was surrounded by a heavy gray mist. I saw an image of Monica as a small child huddled in a corner with no mouth, which I felt symbolized her feeling like she had no voice to express herself.

I explained to Monica what I was seeing, and she confirmed that her mother had passed away as a result of a protracted illness two years previously. Monica had nursed her to the end. Her mother had been a formidable force in Monica's life, dominating and often preventing her from making her own choices.

I asked Monica to thank her mother, say good-bye, and visualize her leaving. I then connected to her mother's energy, and asked her to drop the chain and release Monica, which she did relatively quickly.

Monica's mother then turned around and slowly vanished.

Next, I visualized the harness around Monica's neck falling away and manually unwound the remaining coils of black energy. Clear energy began to flow down through her throat chakra toward her stomach. I removed the chains that were between her throat and sacral chakras.

Next, I saw a large knot of black density lodged in her intestines. I visualized an orange light dissolving the knot until it dissipated and energy flowed down through her intestines. I asked Monica to first imagine orange energy flowing from her head to her feet, spreading beneath her like roots growing into the earth, then red energy flowing back up from the earth and through her body.

After she did that, she could immediately turn her head from side to side and was in slightly less pain. Two weeks later, she called to say that for three days following the healing, she cried incessantly, but the pain in her neck, shoulders, and stomach had gradually subsided and disappeared.

Monica also told me that she now felt a sense of lightness and freedom that she could not remember ever feeling.

6

HOW YOU CAN USE YOUR THOUGHTS AND EMOTIONS TO IMPROVE YOUR HEALTH

How do our thoughts and emotions affect our health?
I am a very emotional person, and I often get overwhelmed by heavy thoughts
and feelings that I don't know how to deal with. Is there a simple process
I can use to release difficult emotions?

I believe that the softest way to heal, although not always easy, is to understand the emotions and energetic patterns stored in your body and then work to release them with ease and grace. By acknowledging your feelings, changing the way you view past traumas, connecting to your inner wisdom, working with Divine Energy, and reprograming your nervous system, you can free yourself from the toxic effects of negative, unconscious beliefs and draining emotions, and embark on a path toward wholeness.

Don't wait until you are sick to start connecting to and listening to your body. I encourage you to create a daily wellness plan that includes meditation, exercise, healthy eating, rest, fun, and laughter. Please refer to the appendix at the end of the book for guidelines on how to create an ongoing life wellness practice.

Emotions and Disease

The link between unresolved negative emotions and disease is undeniable. Scientific research has shown that while negative thoughts, beliefs, attitudes, and emotions weaken the nervous and immune systems, positive emotions release endorphins and build health. Emotions such as depression, fear, anger, disappointment, unworthiness, worry, stress, sadness, hate, jealousy, and irritation can lead to headaches, colds, addiction, allergies, bloating, back pain, asthma, and cancer.

On a physical level, our emotions can literally alter our cell biology and therefore have a profound effect on our well-being. Toxic feelings and thoughts lead to a toxic body, while positive, healthy thoughts and attitudes relax our bodies, giving us more energy and zest for life.

This is not to say that all illness or sickness only comes from emotional issues, or that we can always heal just by dealing with our feelings. There are many different factors that can contribute to someone being unwell, including their environment, genetic predisposition, karma, beliefs, childhood experiences, ancestral and past-life memories, and any unhealthy lifestyle factors, like diet.

The other aspect many people don't take into consideration is that we are energy beings. Though it seems like we only have a physical body, any person trained in the art of intuitive healing knows that we are multidimensional beings with several energy bodies. The energy bodies most easily recognized are the mental, emotional, etheric, and astral, although there are more. Most people have an overdeveloped mental body that contains feelings. Thus, when they are working on their emotions, they may think they are clearing them deeply when, in fact, they are just scratching the surface, changing their thoughts about the emotion rather than releasing the emotion itself. One of the ways to recognize that someone is working on feelings in their mental body is when they say, "I think I felt . . ." When you connect with your emotional body, you know it, as you deeply feel what is going on in your body and your life. You might feel a huge wave of sadness, cry, get angry, feel hurt, or be happy and joyful. The problem is that most people are so uncomfortable with their deepest feelings that they try to do anything they can to suppress and disconnect from the wisdom of their raw emotions.

Your emotional body is strongly linked with your immune, digestive, cardiovascular, and nervous systems. When you push away your emotions, your emotional body can become frozen or torn. If this happens, your immune system becomes greatly weakened, and you are more likely to develop autoimmune problems, inflammation, asthma, lupus, arthritis, and even cancer. You can feel overwhelmed and become extremely tired, sensitive to any type of stress. Your emotional body is your defense system against many illnesses.

You cannot truly let go of your emotions until you feel them fully, and utilize your breath, intention, and possibly touch to release them. There are many wonderful techniques that encourage you to tap, massage, affirm, visualize, move, delete, hum, listen to sounds, and pull out negative emotions from your body. Having been gifted with the capacity to see into the body, I have noticed that when people try to let go of their emotions without feeling the fullness of them, they often cut the ties to and suppress the emotions in their body. This, in turn, creates a tear or a scar in their emotional body, which is extremely sensitive.

It is very important to allow your emotions to come to the surface. This can be done by taking deep breaths, connecting to a particular memory, placing your hand on your body where you feel an emotion, listening to music, or saying a releasing statement aloud. Once the emotion has been fully acknowledged, meaning you have felt it as deeply as possible, you will experience a release of built-up energy. You may even cry and shake or laugh, but it will feel like you are being freed. This is a great time to tap or massage either the point of your body that feels uncomfortable or various points that relate to the issue you are working on. You can then move, shake, dance, or simply sit or lie down to allow your body to complete the process. The most important thing is to listen to your body and go with what it says.

When you read this, please keep in mind that everyone is different, and the best way to heal any challenge is to find a process that resonates with you.

Healing involves looking at your whole life, becoming conscious of what does not work, and fixing it. This may include transforming your point of view, starting to meditate, dealing with unresolved emotional issues, taking supplements, changing your diet, letting go of destructive relationships, changing jobs, and so forth.

Depending on what the physical problem is, you may also need to take medication or have surgery. Even if you have done everything right and surgery is recommended, you should consider it. Certain people may feel that taking medication or having surgery is a failure, but I don't agree. I believe in having a balanced point of view and doing your research. The idea is to be flexible and give yourself the best chance of survival and the highest quality of life, while still participating in your own healing. It is safe to practice healing processes even if you are on medication, as long as you listen to your body and don't overdo anything.

Medication, surgery, and even miracle healing are largely there to buy you time as you discover and work on the real cause of your physical challenge, and change your lifestyle. If you don't, you are highly likely to re-create the illness. Even if doctors can cut out a malignant tumor, they cannot cut energy, which travels through your body impacting the next weakest link.

Humanity's biggest misconception about healing and medical treatments is that most of these treatments have to be tough, violent, and painful. It is generally considered that illness or imbalance in the body is an enemy and that we must attack it in order to destroy it. An important key to healing is perceiving the body as a friend—listening to, understanding, and treating it with gentleness, love, and respect. I believe that the new way of healing is through softness, awareness, and compassion rather than aggression, condemnation, and punishment. As we learn to treat ourselves better, we will also experience a huge change in how we treat each other, our society, and the world.

Scientific Support for Self-Healing

If you need scientific evidence in order to believe that your thoughts, emotions, and behavior can contribute to your illness or health, you can find many studies on the internet and in medical journals that demonstrates this. For instance, the risk of developing heart disease is significantly increased for people who impulsively vent their anger, as well as for those who tend to repress angry feelings.[5]

In a groundbreaking study of 1,200 people at high risk of poor health, it was discovered that those who learned to alter unhealthy mental and emotional attitudes through self-regulation training were more than four times more likely to be alive thirteen years later than an equal-sized control group.[6]

In an article that appeared in the *Journal of Advancement in Medicine*, researchers discovered that heart-focused, sincere, positive feelings boost the immune system, while negative emotions may suppress the immune response for up to six hours following an emotional experience.[7]

Candace Pert, former chief of the Section on Brain Biochemistry of the Clinical Neuroscience Branch at the National Institute of Mental Health and bestselling author of *Molecules of Emotions*, writes, "I've come to believe that virtually all illness, if not psychosomatic in foundation, has a definite psychosomatic component . . . In my talks, I show how the molecules of emotions run every system in our body, and how this communication system is in effect a demonstration of the bodymind's intelligence, an intelligence wise enough to seek wellness, and one that can potentially keep us healthy and disease free without the modern, high-tech medical intervention we now rely on."[8]

Trish's Story: The Body Is the Best Pharmacy

The following is an email I received from Trish, a woman who healed herself by using the processes from my book *The Secret Language of Your Body*:

"I have been suffering from lower back pain for years, trying everything, but nothing worked for very long. My back started to get worse, and I was on painkillers every four hours for a couple of weeks. I would have a week of no pain, and it would all start again.

"I had a scan, and they found a little bit of arthritis in my spine. At this stage, I was desperate, as the medication was damaging my digestive system. I felt depressed and frustrated, being in constant pain, and I felt so old, always waking up stiff.

"I am forty-five years old and the mother of two young boys, so I really wanted to be pain free and flexible. I tried the processes in *The Secret Language of Your Body* and released a lot of stuck emotions.

"The next day, my pain was gone! It was that quick. I have actually started to do squats and sit-ups, something I would have never attempted before because of my troublesome hips and back. And I have had no back pain with my menstruation, which I always dreaded when it was that time of the month. It has been like this now for many months. I don't wake up stiff, and I have saved a lot of money on therapy."

I asked what Trish specifically worked on, and she shared that on the physical level, she did the processes related to the hips and buttocks from *The Secret Language of Your Body*. On the emotional level, she worked on resentment and forgiveness. Although Trish's healing was very quick, I suggest that, for the best results, you regularly work with the emotional release process at the end of this chapter.

Your Body's Innate Intelligence

Deepak Chopra, in his book *Quantum Healing*, states, "The frustrating reality, as far as medical researchers are concerned, is that we already know that the living body is the best pharmacy ever devised. It produces diuretics, painkillers, tranquilizers, sleeping pills, antibiotics, and indeed everything manufactured by the drug companies, but it makes them much, much better. The dosage is always right and given on time; side effects are minimal or nonexistent; and the directions for using the drug are included in the drug itself, as part of its built-in intelligence."[9]

The reason the above statement may not seem true to most people is because they have not been taught how to tune in to their body and communicate with it in an effective way—that allows it to access its own healing potential.

We can all discover how to access the body's innate intelligence to heal ourselves while using medicine when it is appropriate. I have worked with and led workshops with doctors who practice integrative medicine. Whenever I have tuned in to a client and felt that there could be a possibility of a serious problem, I have always encouraged him or her to consult with a doctor and get tests, as I believe there is a place for medicine and self-healing: the former can save lives, and be extremely helpful short term and, at times, long term—especially when people have no understanding of how to illicit healing experiences from their own body, or simply don't have enough energy to heal themselves.

However, since so many drugs have very unpleasant side effects, learning how to heal yourself should be a necessity for all!

Patrick Quanten writes, "Illnesses are not the result of a vicious attack by an outside aggressor but are internal imbalances. Bugs appear in diseased tissues from within the tissues itself, as has been demonstrated in laboratory conditions. There are no mysterious viruses that travel vast distances or lie dormant for decades before 'attacking' the innocent victim. Illness has not so much to do with 'out there' as it has with 'in here.' It is an internal affair and should therefore be treated as one. What is required is a shift in thinking. We need to stop blaming outside factors for internal problems. We need to regard the whole rather than the parts as the essence of life."[10]

Emotional healing requires you to tune in and become aware of unresolved emotions that are stuck in your body, to recognize them, to feel them, and to let them go. When an emotion or experience that has created change and limitation in your life is transformed, you will feel lighter, look softer, and allow new, more empowering opportunities to come into your life. Your body will also have access to new healing and revitalizing energy that can help you restore your body to better health.

To experience emotional healing, you need to make a commitment to succeed by taking responsibility for your actions and reactions. Taking responsibility does not mean blaming yourself for being unwell; on the contrary, it means discovering the decisions you made that did not work, changing your perspective, and moving forward. Take a moment now to think about a difficult time in your life and ask, *What have I learned? What would I do differently?*

Healing yourself by learning to tune in to your body, emotions, and spirit, gives you an opportunity to forgive yourself and others, let go of past hurts, clear blocks, and awaken aspects of yourself that you were unaware of. It puts you in the driver's seat and allows for self-discovery. When taking a healing approach, I encourage you to view your body as an intelligent force that, when guided correctly, has the power to regenerate.

Healing does not only affect physical well-being; it can also enhance relationships, help you find your life purpose, increase finances, expand spiritual awareness, and bring peace, fulfillment, and confidence to your life.

Changing Your Thoughts and Emotions

I have spent many years researching how thoughts and emotions affect the body and how to deal with them. From my experience, the body will follow your instructions. If you constantly say that you can't handle things, your hands may become stiff and clenched, and you won't be able to handle anything new. If you consistently say, for example, "My boss is a pain in the neck," you may manifest neck problems. When you think, *Oh, what a headache this will be*, your body listens. Because it is good at taking directions, it immediately starts building tension and pain in your head.

Dr. Robin Youngson, founder of the Centre for Compassion in Healthcare, says, "*Livid, pissed off, torn up inside, heartache, bone weary, jaundiced, gut wrenching, blood boiling, pain in the neck, stab in the back, takes my breath away, a rash decision, sick to death*—our language is alive with ancient wisdom about the origin of many illnesses."[11]

Your nervous system is the primary system in your body, which acts as your faithful servant, learning from your beliefs, words, behaviors, and reactions to outside stimuli, as well as from your environment and the people you closely associate with. Then it applies what it has discovered to your body, organs, and overall wellness. In fact, the nervous system pretty much looks for role models to mimic. This is great if you associate with healthy, empowered people who encourage and up lift you. However, it presents challenges if you are surrounded by extremely critical and fearful company.

In order to really transform your health, you need to learn not only to refocus your mind and release unhealthy emotions but also to reprogram your nervous system. I encourage anyone who has a serious medical condition to practice the healing processes from my book *The Secret Language of Your Body*, as well as this book, and to regularly implement the nervous system process in order to condition the body to be well. In fact, even if you are well, I encourage you to work regularly with your nervous system. I include a short process of expanding your nervous system in chapter 18, "How You Can Create More Money and Success in Your Life" (see page 231). However, if you are working on your health (versus your finances), you might want to use the nervous system exercise from *The Secret Language of Your Body*.

Valerie's Story: Releasing Stagnant Emotions

For several months, Valerie had a chest infection and a cough that she could not get rid of. She tried everything possible, but nothing worked. While sitting in a cafe, Valerie was flipping through a magazine on natural health when she came upon an article I had written on tuning in to your body and releasing stuck emotions. Valerie followed the process described and discovered that she was carrying feelings of deep rejection, criticism, and judgment from when she was a teenager.

The next day, Valerie bought my book and worked with the emotional processes. By the following day, her cough had disappeared.

Petrea King, founding director of the Quest for Life Centre, says, "Our issues are in our tissues. When we react to people or events in our lives, we literally re-activate a physiology in our body that we have experienced before."[12] Deep insight and acknowledgement of what has been stuck in your body allows for a profound transformation as you let go of painful points of view you have been carrying. For instance, although Valerie may not have been conscious that she was holding on to rejection and criticism from her school days, her body was carrying cellular memories of being bullied. Her persistent cough was a way to make her pay attention and discover how her old, painful experiences were affecting the quality of her life. When I questioned Valerie, she revealed that she still felt nervous about speaking up and sharing her opinion for fear of being judged. This was a huge drawback, as Valerie had a home business in which she needed to use her communication skills to attract clients.

I encouraged Valerie to connect with her inner teenager every day for a week, surrounding her with love, support, and affection. I also suggested that she work on her self-esteem and nervous system. Within a month, Valerie's business doubled, and she felt more confident, especially about her ability to express herself. The next time I saw her, I noticed that she looked younger and more relaxed. Valerie shared that after many years of restless sleep, she was finally able to sleep well.

I believe Valerie was able to have a more restful sleep because she was no longer on guard, subconsciously trying to protect herself from being attacked. She felt safe, and thus was able to relax, move forward, and grow. And this, in turn, attracted positive people to her.

Go to this link to learn more about my self-healing journey. It reveals many important factors about healing and what is possible.

http://innasegal.com/the-secret-of-life-wellness-downloads/my-self-healing-journey

Process for Releasing Emotions

When you discover a stuck emotion in your body, you can use the following emotional healing process to help release it. If there is pain in an area of your body, discomfort, or any type of physical disturbance, then there is often an underlying, challenging experience or emotion that is stored in the cells of your body. The best way to stay healthy is to focus on releasing a negative emotion or a hurtful experience, either immediately after it has occurred or within twenty-four hours of it occurring. While you may not be able to change what you have done in the past, you can certainly influence your present and future well-being!

Connect with and Explore Your Emotions

Place your hands on the part of your body where you feel a dense, heavy emotion most intensely. Be aware that there are often several emotions piled on top of each other. When you become conscious of one, others may also surface. Concentrate on the strongest one for now.

Breathe into that area slowly and deeply, allowing any emotion to rise to the surface with as little resistance as possible.

If you are having difficulty accessing your feelings, it is extremely useful to play some appropriate music. If you are feeling sad, a stirring slow song will help you connect to your sadness and grief. If you are feeling angry, play a louder, faster song. Tune in to your body to see if you feel like moving; movement can greatly help release emotions. Your movements may be very soft and flowing or very sharp and fast.

Explore where this emotion comes from. Ask yourself: *Is this feeling related to what I am experiencing at present, or is it connected to the past? What is my earliest memory of feeling this emotion? What happened? What decision did I make about myself, my life, and what I am capable of creating? Is this my feeling, or did I observe someone who was close to me exhibiting it and then assume it as my own? Am I willing to let it go and free myself?*

Say a Clearing Statement

Repeat the following statement with feeling and a strong intention to heal: "Divine Healing Intelligence, using the orange-red flame of purification, please dissolve any destructive, limiting, and stagnant emotions from my cellular memories, such as ____ _____." (State the emotions you would like to work on. It is preferable to work on either one specific emotion or several that are related.)

Take some deep breaths and allow any dense, destructive, and limiting emotions to be released. You may visualize heavy, smoky energy coming out of your body or feel stress and tension leaving your body. It doesn't matter what the image or sensation is, just allow it to release, and keep breathing until you feel freer. If you feel comfortable, you can place your hands just above or next to the area you are working on; then imagine drawing out negative energy (that may look like gray or black clouds) from your body with your hands. Afterward, shake out your hands as you imagine placing all this old, stagnant energy into a purple flame and watching it burn away.

Say: "Divine Healing Intelligence, please help me release limited points of view and let go of all inflexibility in my mind, body, and emotions."

Take some more deep breaths and soften your body. Become aware of any areas of your body where you feel emotions, and tap on or massage this area.

Say: "Divine Wisdom, work with me to release any patterns of strain, struggle, and resistance."

Allow your Divine Intelligence to wash away all strain, struggle, and resistance.

Say: "Please dissolve any blockages in my mind, body, and emotions that obstruct my flow of energy and circulation. Thank you."

Allow yourself to connect to the soulful part of you that can dissolve and wash away all blockages.

Now repeat the word "CLEAR" several times. Relax your fingers and hands, and then shake them for twenty to thirty seconds while taking slow, deep breaths. Focus on letting go of stress and heaviness from your body.

Perform a Mudra

Mudras are healing hand gestures that help you to connect to your breath and release stagnant energy while revitalizing your body. They are simple and effortless. One of their biggest functions is to release stress. Below is a powerful mudra to help you to let go of any challenging emotions that remain.

Sit or stand with your spine straight. Take some deep breaths through your nose, and breathe out through your mouth. Touch your thumbs with your index fingers, and extend the rest of your fingers. Place your right arm at the level of your heart, with your thumb and index finger pointing down. Place your left arm at the level of your solar plexus with the thumb and the index finger pointing up and touching the thumb and the index fingers of your right arm.

Hum the sound *aum* for forty seconds to several minutes (for this process, *au* is pronounced like the *o* in *home*). This mudra helps you to balance your yin and yang energies, while the sound *aum* helps to clear all the stuckness and bring your vibration up toward Divinity.

Visualize an orange-red flame moving through your body, mind, emotions, and energy field. If you have difficulty visualizing, you may consider working with my card deck on color healing, *The Secret Language of Color Cards*, by looking at a red and an orange card. Observe or sense as your Divine Intelligence dissolves all negative thoughts, words, feelings, memories, and images associated with a particular person, place, or experience that has bound you.

PART II

MASTERING YOUR SOUL'S JOURNEY

As you learn to go within, to discover how to love all the various shadow and light aspects of yourself, and to work on your energy centers, emotions, and stress levels, you become ready to discover more about your soul's journey, and how you can align with and reach your highest potential. In this section, you will connect to your soul and rediscover its language.

As karma is mentioned several times throughout this section, it is important to clarify that I consider karma to be unresolved energy that has been carried from the past, including other lives and dimensions. Karma is considered to be the "law of cause and effect" that requires us to take responsibility for our actions and our reactions. Some karma is connected to our unfulfilled desires, keeping us attached to our limitations. We can dissolve a lot of karma when we evolve, make positive healing choices, fully learn and integrate our lessons, become more compassionate, and bring light and love to others. In this sense, what we do to others, we do unto ourselves.

7

How You Can Connect and Communicate with Your Soul

What exactly is your definition of a soul, and how do I connect to my soul and communicate with it? Also, can I ask my soul for guidance?

Your soul is the most eternal part of you; it is an aspect of Divinity. The soul enters your body during gestation and leaves your body when you die. The soul is a Divine, intelligent entity that resides with other souls in the spirit world. It learns, grows, and evolves both in the spirit world and the physical world. Part of your soul's energy always stays in the spirit world and is connected to Divinity. This part remains pure and whole even if an aspect of the soul that has come to earth becomes affected by density, negativity, heavy karma, or difficult experiences. People often refer to this part of you as your Higher Self.

Your soul has chosen to have different experiences in a human form in order to expand, learn important lessons, resolve karmic energy, be of service, and evolve.

Your role on this planet is to also love, share, and impact and connect with other souls. As you reconnect with important people in your life, you can heal past pain, reclaim your innate gifts and abilities, and support, encourage, and inspire each other to be your best.

The Soul's Journey: Finding Our Highest Role

From years of working with people, I have realized that there are two points of view that we can live our lives from. The first is based on safety and survival of the physical, and the second is focused on the spiritual journey and intention of the soul.

Many people I have met live their lives largely based on survival. They are taught the importance of having a nice family, a good house, and a job that is safe and pays the bills. They are encouraged to please their relatives, and adapt to the rules and beliefs of the society they live in. Most have disconnected from their heart and the true desire of their soul, allowing predictability and the need for physical security to rule their lives. They have forgotten to listen to their heart, take risks, and discover their inner treasures.

This is not to say that your soul does not desire you to be safe and supported in your life. But it's your soul that knows your true potential, abilities, and opportunities. From your childhood, your soul tries to grab your attention by giving you creative ideas, feelings of excitement, and intuitive guidance. It wants to lead you into the most exciting, joyous, and expansive experience of your life. Your soul knows that you are an unlimited being of light, capable of great feats of courage, deep love, healing, and creativity. It recognizes your capacity for greatness and evolution, and that understands that you are an important key in the wheel of life, your choices influence the world.

We are all like waves in the big ocean of life, affecting each other through our thoughts, words, feelings, actions, vibrations, and interactions with each other. As technology advances, we benefit by having enhanced opportunities to touch each other's lives. Our highest role is to reconnect with the power of Divinity, raise our vibration, move toward being in tune with our deepest guidance, and create a ripple effect of healing throughout the world. Each of us has an enormous capacity to live consciously, joyously, and abundantly, regardless of our circumstances.

Before your soul comes into the physical, it has an awareness of what you are capable of achieving in the body in the time period you have chosen, and with the people who surround you. Even if it seems random to you now, your soul has chosen this experience from a deep understanding of how everything in your life is set up—to give you the opportunity to grow, learn, and live your life's purpose.

Don't Let Your Rational Mind Stop You from Living Your Soul Purpose

The biggest blockades that stop you from living your soul purpose are fear and linear thinking. Your soul does not function on the level of the mind. It operates on the vibrational level of higher wisdom, feelings, sensations, and intuition. It can understand things the rational mind does not—that everything is possible if it is in your soul path and is for the highest good of all, even miracles! *A Course in Miracles* states that "There is no order of difficulty in miracles. One is not 'harder' or 'bigger' than another. They are all the same."[13] Your soul knows that even what your mind would deem impossible is possible and can occur.

The challenge is to not overuse the mind for the matters of the heart and the soul. This does not mean that the mind is useless. In fact, it can be extremely helpful in understanding ideas, performing certain actions, and taking care of everyday life. The problem occurs when the mind takes over, and you no longer feel happy, joyful, and alive. You become a judging, controlling, doing machine, rather than a living, breathing, evolving spirit.

Soul Communication: How to Hear What Your Soul Is Telling You

In order to have great health, you need to learn how to communicate with your body. To create nourishing relationships, you have to express yourself in ways that others understand and that inspire them to offer their love and support. Deep fulfillment in your life is tied to recognizing and achieving your soul purpose. This is the next level of knowing yourself, strengthening your ability to commune with the Divine, and becoming con-scious of your internal and external guidance system.

I have had so many amazing, miraculous experiences in my life that I can't deny I am truly guided. I regularly ask my soul to assist me in making my dreams a reality, and to help me grow, transform, and evolve.

Most people don't ask their hearts for what they truly desire because they are scared that their hearts will come up with something unrealistic. However, what most people don't realize is that even if you think you are too old to start dancing, acting, singing, or pursuing some other creative venture, your soul might be guiding you to meet someone in that singing class, dancing class, or spiritual retreat—someone who will give you the guidance, skills, or ideas you need to move toward discovering your soul purpose.

The important thing is to listen to and follow your guidance.

When you finally decide to communicate with your soul, it will give you direction through strong feelings, thoughts, visions, books, desires, dreams, other people, signs, songs, teachers, and any other ways that it can reach you. Your soul communicates most often through feelings and sensations; for instance, your heart may beat faster, you may feel a tingling sensation and receive an image, you may remember something important, or you may just know what to do next.

You can also receive messages from your soul by paying attention to your heart's desires, intuitions, dreams, visions, and synchronicities. You may meet a person you have not seen for years who has an answer to a question you have; a song may come on the radio that has a verse you need to hear; someone may send you an email with information you are looking for; or a book may fall off a shelf in a bookstore that has the solution you need.

Your biggest task is to ask questions, relax, and meditate so that you can become more sensitive, to listen to and follow your soul's guidance. Be open, pay attention, and follow the signs. The most wonderful thing about this awareness is the knowledge that you are loved, guided, and supported.

My Story: My Deepest Longing

Since I was a child, my deepest longing was to become an actress. Whenever I thought about acting, my heart would beat faster, my energy would heighten, and my passion would explode. Anyone who knew me understood that my heart was set on being a performer.

I loved the idea of experiencing life from different perspectives and knew that through drama, I could develop a deeper understanding of other people, myself, and the world around me. However, when I turned fourteen, all the students at my school had to attend career days, where people from different industries would share their experiences.

Whenever I mentioned what I wanted to do, I heard big sighs and was told that there was no work or money in acting. After a lot of discouragement and negativity, I decided to focus my attention on something that could give me better job opportunities. I settled on copywriting, as it was creative, respected, and well paid. When my mother told me she thought I should be a pharmacist, which seemed like a good, secure job, I just laughed and told her that it might be her dream but it was not mine.

Not long after making the decision to give up on acting, an interesting phenomenon began to occur: I started to wake between 5 and 6 in the morning with the most overwhelming desire to act. The more I tried to suppress it, the stronger it became. After a few months of enduring this, I knew that I needed to do something creative to calm myself.

I decided to attend a dance class. There, I met Jane, a twenty-six-year-old medical student. Jane gave me a book titled *Born to Succeed*. This book was my first introduction to spirituality and the idea that we are cocreators of our dreams. Not long after I started reading this book, something incredible happened. I was sitting in my study, gazing through my window, when I had a vision. I saw myself sitting on top of a mountain, speaking to thousands of people. I experienced a deep, profound love and appreciation that flowed from me to them and from them to me. Even though I could not understand the meaning of this vision, I knew that I was receiving a message from a higher source.

The day after my vision, I woke earlier than usual with an even greater desire to act. No matter what I tried to do that day, I could not suppress it. It was as if I was having an internal battle. That night, when I came home, I picked up *Born to Succeed* and asked my soul to show me what it wanted me to understand. I closed my eyes, opened the book at random, and placed my finger in the middle of a page. Opening my eyes, I read, "God wants you to do what you want to do." These words touched a deep place inside my being.

I began reflecting on the fact that I wanted to study acting from my heart and soul, even though most of my friends cringed at the idea of acting in plays and movies (their worst nightmare). I also realized that my desire to act was not intellectual; the more I tried to use my mind to suppress it, the more my inner yearning to perform awakened. I understood that, like most people, I had thought that I needed to please my parents and teachers, and do what they thought was best for me. However, in that moment, I realized that my own soul and Divine Intelligence would not give me the desire to act if it was not part of my soul purpose. I made an instant decision to enroll myself in an acting class.

The next morning, I woke, feeling lively and enthusiastic but peaceful. I told my mum what I wanted to do and spent the day inquiring about acting classes. Deep inside, I felt that my soul was leading me to my real life's work. Those classes changed my life and helped prepare me for eventually teaching people to heal and transform their lives.

From my very first acting class, I felt my soul soar, like I was given wings to fly. Through the training, I became more mature, understanding, and compassionate. I learned leadership qualities, decision making, and more than anything, trust. Intuitively, I knew that in the class, I would meet the person I needed to share my life with. Although it did not happen instantly, within a year of doing the class, I met my husband, Paul.

While I did not become a traditional actress like I had dreamed when I was younger, following my internal guidance has led me to do the most incredibly rewarding work, which is to help people heal their bodies and transform their lives. Interestingly, on my journey, I have hosted a television and radio show, presented segments on different television programs, and have been interviewed in many countries all over the world. I always seem to be working on interesting television and film projects. So, the television and acting training I received has definitely been helpful.

In my acting classes, I experienced exploration, playfulness, and fun. Through my courses, I try to demonstrate to others that transformation may be challenging, but it is also fun, joyful, and incredibly rewarding.

Soul Agreements

Soul agreements are often made by your soul before you incarnate. They can direct you toward your soul mates, the situations you need to heal, and your life purpose. Soul agreements can also help you release or balance your karmic patterns from previous lives (as well as your current life) and evolve. Major experiences in your life—ones that make you stop and change your path—could be predestined. This can include accidents, diseases, big losses, surprising job offers, or trips to significant places that change your life direction. You may also have an agreement to meet soul mates, life partners, teachers, and enlightened masters.

At times, your soul agreement could be to learn kindness, lead by example, create a painting, write a book or a movie, or just makes a difference. Thus, developing your intuition and listening to your inner calling, as well as recurring external signs, can be a way that your soul is urging you to move forward.

Dr. Caroline Myss is a pioneer in the field of energy medicine and human consciousness, a world renowned lecturer, a medical intuitive, and a bestselling author. When I interviewed her, she shared:

> My work on sacred contracts has to do with exploring the idea that each one of us has a collection of agreements we have made before we were born, and that each of these agreements or contracts determines the way our life plays out, who we meet, our opportunities and challenges. It does not determine the outcome—this is where choice comes in. It does predetermine that there are people you will meet, opportunities that will come to you. How you respond

when you meet these people or engage in the opportunity is fully and totally in your hands, and this is where self-esteem and choice come in.[14]

It's important to recognize that we can also make vows and soul agreements in our daily lives. And these agreements can often create an unexpected and profound effect on our long-term experiences.

I have had some clients who have made soul agreements that have taken them toward their greatest fulfillment, and others who have made agreements that have caused them a lot of pain and suffering because they did not understand the power of those agreements. If you make a vow or soul agreement, please take it seriously and work toward fulfilling it if it is still for your greatest good. Alternatively, release it with ease and grace if you have grown beyond it. You can begin by becoming aware of your agreements and asking Divine Intelligence to help you fulfill them or let them go, if they are no longer serving you.

Go to this link to read an amazing story about Michael J. Roads and a soul agreement he made that challenged him to his core and completely transformed his reality.
http://innasegal.com/the-secret-of-life-wellness-downloads/michaels-story

Processes for Connecting to Your Soul

In order to increase your connection to your soul, you need to have time to relax and meditate. Sit on a chair or sit cross-legged. Focus on your body, and become aware of what you feel inside. Take slow, deep breaths with the intention of being open to your own Divinity and Soul Communication.

Hold a mudra by touching your index fingers together and your thumbs together while interlocking the rest of your fingers. Your index fingers should be facing upward toward your head and your thumbs downward toward your feet. Hold this posture in front of your heart, with your elbows pointing out to the sides. Focus your attention on connecting to your soul energy and receiving guidance. If you could feel or imagine the energy of your soul, what would it be like? Allow yourself to meditate on this. If your soul had a color, what color would it be? When you sense the color, imagine it bathing your whole body.

Say: "Divine Healing Intelligence, please help me to deeply reconnect with my soul and my heart's desires. Allow me to become more open to the messages and guidance from my soul. Give me the ability to listen to my soul and allow it to heal any pain, struggle, or sabotage in my life. Allow me to experience my highest good and follow my life's Divine plan. Reveal to me the blessings, opportunities, joy, happiness, and abundance that await me as I follow my soul journey. Thank you."

Repeat the word "CLEAR" several times, until you feel lighter.

Relax your hands and allow yourself to soften even further. As you take a slow breath in, focus your attention above your head. Imagine gold light pouring into your head, moving into your throat. As you breathe out, feel the energy release from your heart, expanding outward. Repeat this five times.

Place your hands on your heart. Ask what your heart and soul really desire, then pay attention. If an answer comes, write it down. Ask your soul to show you what steps you need to take to achieve this desire or bring it into your reality. If you do not receive any answers, be patient; your soul knows that you have begun the process of connecting and listening to it, and will start to give you answers as you open up more and more.

Whenever you have a question, ask your soul for guidance, then allow the answers to either arise in yourself or be shown to you in time.

8

How You Can Connect to Divine Energy and Protect Yourself

*When I walk into a room full of people, I feel like I pick up their energy,
and then I feel unwell. I've heard that it's really helpful to do a process
of connecting to Divine Energy and protecting yourself.
Could you expand on that and explain how to do it?*

Most people can relate to having gone into a room, house, or building and feeling a sensation of heaviness or stagnation, and then visiting another space and feeling lighter, brighter, and more peaceful. When you walk into a house where people have had an argument or feel upset or angry, you can often sense that all is not well. If you are sensitive or feel weak, it is likely that those negative vibrations will affect you and make you unwell.

You may not be aware of how those energies have entered your space and intertwined around your own energy field, yet you may become conscious of suddenly feeling weary, drained, and lackluster. Certain individuals can experience internal coldness, numbness, heaviness, tension, and depression in a space that is energetically polluted. Others may find it difficult to breathe or move, get stomach bloating, or experience pain or headaches.

When I began to learn about healing, I realized how easy it was to pick up dense or heavy energies from other people. When I teach, I often explain that part of my

111

own sickness occurred because I always listened to other people's problems, and then absorbed their emotional and physical pain into my body. Thus, I often felt achy after having a conversation with someone who was going through a challenging time.

Protecting Your Energy

At times, I've heard theories that protection is a fear-based belief and that there is nothing to fear. Since I don't like buying into fear, I decided to experiment by not protecting myself for six months.

During those six months, I constantly got colds and felt unwell. In fact, one day I felt so horrible that I was throwing up. Thinking that I had been poisoned, I made an appointment to see a naturopath who was also a spiritual healer. When I came into his office, he asked me to lie down on the massage table. After checking my energy, he told me that I had picked up too much of other people's negative energy and that my body could not handle it. Thus, I was literally vomiting it out. He told me that if I wanted to be well, I needed to protect myself.

I realized then that protection does not have to be about fear but about purification, clarity, and vibrational cleanliness. When I learned to connect to Divine Healing Intelligence and protect my own space, I was able to listen to other people's problems without being physically drained or affected. Interestingly, the times I forgot to protect myself when I worked with a client, I felt weak, tense, and exhausted. It did not help me or anyone I was working with to take on their negative energy and store it in my body. I realized that the clearer I was, and the more connected I was to Divinity, the more I could help others and the healthier I would be.

Another way to look at it is to think of wearing clothes. If it's really sunny outside, you might apply some sunscreen and wear a hat to protect yourself. If it is cold and rainy, you might wear a coat and take an umbrella so you don't get wet.

Lawrence's Story: Maintaining His Own Energy

Lawrence owned his own business, and by the end of each day, he was always so exhausted that it was difficult to have a conversation with him.

I told him that even though I understood the stress of owning a business, being so exhausted was not normal for a thirty-year-old man.

Lawrence was constantly surrounded by people who wanted things from him. It occurred to me that his exhaustion related to needing to please others. After a full day of work his shoulders were hunched, his face pale, and his eyes looked puffy. I taught Lawrence to protect himself by encouraging him to do the connection to the Divine and protection process in the morning and at lunchtime.

A week later, I met Lawrence at a dinner party. At 10 PM, he seemed bright, energetic, and lively. He told me that he had followed my advice and was feeling fantastic. He said he could not remember the last time he had so much energy. He also told me that his clients seemed a lot less needy and draining, and that he was actually enjoying his work, instead of being frustrated or stressed.

A Powerful Way to Start Your Day

I encourage everyone I teach to begin their day by connecting to Divine Energy, protecting themselves and setting their intention for the day. This process not only strengthens your energy field and protects you from picking up other people's pain and tension, but it also helps you to have more clarity, courage, and motivation. Consistent use of this process will help you connect to, listen to, and trust your intuition.

My intention is to help you focus your attention on having the greatest day possible, performing your actions from a place of relaxation, compassion, and love. The feedback that I have received from thousands of people who have practiced this process is that they feel clearer, purer, and more connected to Divinity. They also feel comfortable walking into rooms full of people or going to places that have heavy or dense vibrations, knowing they will still feel good.

For the people who are in healing professions, whether you are a doctor, healer, nurse, chiropractor, or practitioner of any other wellness modality, it is really important to do this process before you see each client, even if you have only time for the last part.

This process also helps protect you from other people's aggression and negativity. The more you can hold your own clear energy, the healthier you will be.

Process for Protecting and Purifying Your Energy

I suggest you do this process several times each day, especially when you are around negative, needy, or draining people.

Brilliant white and gold are powerful colors that you can use to connect to the Divine. White, the color of purity, is great for clearing toxicity and dense energy from the body. Brilliant white intensifies the purifying energy of ordinary white, thus dissolving density faster. Gold helps heal stress, trauma, frustration, aggression, depression, and illness. Combining gold and brilliant white makes this process more powerful.

Protect and Purify

First, open your palms (so that they are facing up) to send the message to Universal Intelligence that you are ready to receive. Take some slow, deep breaths. Allow your body to soften and relax. Imagine that you are showered with rays of brilliant white and gold light.

Say: "Divine Source, I ask that you surround me with your rays of brilliant white and gold light, moving through my whole body, energy field, mind, and emotions. Please purify my mind, emotions, body, and energy field. Release any confusion in my mind about what actions I need to take today and replace it with clarity, courage, and motivation to do my best, for the highest good of all."

Take a few deep breaths while saying the word "CLEAR" to let go of any confusion about what you need to do that day.

Say: "Divine Wisdom, help me acknowledge the feelings that come from my heart, soul, and intuition and to become aware of their messages. Allow me to listen to my Higher Self and live this day in a truthful, courageous, and empowered manner. Help me to recognize and handle any resistance, self-sabotage, or negativity in the most appropriate and loving ways. Help me release any mental overwhelm, internal conflict, density, and heaviness that may be present in my mind, body, or emotions."

Take a few deep breaths while saying the word "CLEAR" to let go of any confusion about what you need to do that day.

Say: "Divine Source, please bring lightness into my body, allowing me to expand and open myself to the wonderful new possibilities and opportunities that this day may bring. Please protect me from picking up any density and negativity from other beings, which is not mine and has nothing to do with me. Allow me to have compassion without the need to carry other people's burdens. Thank You."

Repeat the word "CLEAR" several times, until your feel lighter.

Note that if you have limited time or you are doing the process more than once a day, you can just do the last part of the process above, starting with "Divine Source."

Imagine brilliant white and gold rays of light bathing you, healing you, and clearing all density, negativity, distrust, limitation, and pain out of your body and energy field.

9

HOW YOU CAN EXPERIENCE UNCONDITIONAL LOVE

How do I experience unconditional love for others?

Wouldn't it be amazing to be surrounded by people with whom you could be your true self and share what you were thinking or feeling without being afraid that they would stop loving you, even if they disagree or have a different point of view? Wouldn't you love to communicate with people on the level of their hearts and souls, where you feel safe to share your deepest, most intimate feelings and thoughts?

Unconditional love requires softness, forgiveness, and an ability to love the other person no matter how they behave. It involves wisdom, patience, and maturity to be who you are, without the need to please others, while allowing others to be who they are. When we stop seeking or giving others approval, we offer them the most amazing opportunity to grow and expand. By releasing our ideas, beliefs, and expectations of who they are, we allow them to discover who they are.

The trick is to be loving, caring, and helpful without being attached to an outcome. To experience unconditional love, we need to stop putting expectations on our love. This means loving people for who they are, not who we would like them to be.

The Challenges of Unconditional Love

The biggest missing pieces in conditional love are a lack of communication and a willingness to listen, understand, and see other points of view. Often, there is a sense of self-righteousness, where one or both parties feel that they are correct or justified in treating the other poorly. It is easy to judge people's behavior and then withdraw our love, support, and affection when they do not do what we want them to. This is love with strings attached, which contains an element of threat. Instead of focusing on ourselves, it is easier to focus on how others' behavior makes us feel uncomfortable, unpleasant, and challenged, and then blame them. It is even easier to punish them by sulking, guilt-tripping, becoming cold, disconnecting, or shutting down.

Laura's Story: Strings Attached

Laura realized that she was gay when she was fifteen. Her parents were from a Greek, religious background and felt ashamed of Laura's sexual preference, even though Laura was extremely intelligent, hardworking, and easygoing. When Laura was in her early twenties, her parents proposed to buy her a house if she promised to stop being intimate with women. When Laura refused, they told her that they would not offer her any more financial or emotional assistance, and that she was on her own.

Laura was so distraught that she began to develop an eating disorder, eventually ending up in the hospital. For Laura, her parents' approval was so important that she could not digest her food or stomach her life. After a lot of healing and self-development work, Laura realized that she had to forgive and love her parents despite their views and behavior.

As Laura transformed and stopped trying to get parental approval for her life preferences, her parents began to soften their opinions and relax. They even started inviting Laura and her female partner to their house. Although Laura's relationship with her parents has improved dramatically, she says that moving toward unconditional love is a daily practice.

Consideration for Imperfection

It is important to understand that being able to share with others doesn't mean saying or doing hurtful things to test their love; it means taking people into consideration and finding ways to express your feelings in a loving, compassionate manner. You have to recognize that neither you nor others are perfect. Salvador Dali famously said, "Have no fear of perfection—you'll never reach it." Some people consider perfectionism to be a mental illness that needs to be cured with courage, faith, and a desire to serve others from your heart. We are all in the process of learning, so self-forgiveness, as well as acknowledging where you may have said or done something hurtful, is crucial.

One of the most beautiful experiences in life is to be accepted and loved for who you are, with all of your idiosyncrasies and imperfections. I have talked, taught, and written about the shadow side because everybody can relate to this. A few years ago, I was discussing different aspects of the shadow with a close friend when he averted his eyes and shamefully admitted that he can be very selfish and self-centered. I smiled at him and replied, "I know, and I still love you just as much." When he heard that, his whole posture changed, and I could see that he felt safe to express and love himself.

Unconditional love is a way of life. It requires an understanding that everyone is free to learn and grow from their own experiences. Sometimes they will choose to listen to you, and at other times they will follow their own guidance. Sometimes they will make mistakes, and at other times they will triumph. Loving without conditions is a moment-by-moment experience that helps us explore where we feel free in our lives, as well as the areas we need to work on.

My Story: Practicing Unconditional Love

I met my husband Paul when I was eighteen years old, and he shared various ideas about unconditional love with me. He told me that he used to practice seeing everyone as beautiful beings of light when traveling on the bus or walking. I noticed that wherever we went, people seemed to like and accept him, even when he would say strange things or behave in unconventional ways.

At the time when I met Paul, I had a very challenging relationship with my father, whom I judged harshly and who I felt was making my life unbearable. In fact, I was so enraged by my father's choices and behavior that I had stopped talking to him. One day, while sitting in my parent's back garden, I bitterly complained to Paul about my dad. After listening for a while, Paul said, "You really feel like you are a victim don't you?" I told him that in this situation, I definitely felt helpless and like a victim.

Paul asked me if I enjoyed being in this situation. I told him that I felt I had no choice. He inquired if I was open to healing my relationship with my father. I told him that, although I could not see how, I was willing to try anything. Paul asked me to imagine my dad in front of me. He then invited me to see past all the appearances and behaviors I did not like, and become aware of who my dad really was.

As Paul was guiding me, I felt my consciousness begin to shift. I saw my father's soul and was completely taken aback, as I had never seen a soul before. Dad's soul shining in front of me was pure, Divine, and loving, and I felt deeply touched by the healing energy I felt from this recognition. Instantly, I realized that my dad was not his behavior, his beliefs, or his actions; his soul was bright, loving, and soft. I felt all my judgments, opinions, and righteousness melt away. It was as if, on the conscious level, we were playing a tug of war. I was pulling the rope one way, and he was pulling it the other. When I saw the truth of who my dad really is, I let go of the rope. Something deep and profound had shifted inside me.

That day, when my dad came home, he gave me a big hug, told me how much he loved me, and asked me to forgive him. I was so touched, I cried. This happened without me saying a word about my experience. From the moment I saw my dad's soul, our relationship healed and transformed from conditional to unconditional love.

Interestingly, there have been several times since when I did not agree with my father's choices or behaviors but felt that who he really is factors in so much more importantly than what he does. I have not felt the need to judge, punish, or be upset with him. Instead, I take the time to explain my point of view, without making him feel like he is wrong, and he has done the same with me when I have gone through challenging times.

To love someone irrespective of their choices and behavior is unbelievably liberating.

Unconditional Love as a Higher Level of Consciousness

Unconditional Love can also be seen as a higher state of consciousness—one in which you are not focused on your own selfish needs, points of view, or desires. You love because that is who you are; you give because giving, caring, and supporting is your natural state. This love is not romantic or controlled by desire, neediness, or eroticism. It's pure, intuitive, inclusive, compassionate, devotional, and freeing.

This kind of unconditional love is aligned with Divinity and thus is holy, sacred, and nonlinear. From this position, there is no jealousy or need for ownership, and a person has the capacity to deeply love many people at the same time. Here, a person looks at life from a higher spiritual perspective, and the love they feel is consistent and independent of external factors and conditions. Love becomes a way of living and relating to everyone and everything. The world also becomes illuminated by beauty, synchronicity, and grace.

While some people are born into this vibration of unconditional love and therefore see the world from an enlightened perspective, others have to work toward evolving to a space of unconditional love by facing their shadow, transcending their pain, and connecting to their Divinity.

I met an extraordinary man called Reverend Nirvana, who experienced the Divinity of love while being held at gunpoint. The love he felt was so dazzling that his attacker withdrew the gun from near his head, turned away, and left him alone.

At one point in his life, Reverend Nirvana meditated on experiencing the depths, essence, and power of love every day for an entire year, until he could maintain a consistent inner experience of love and joy regardless of outer circumstances. He powerfully emanates and expresses this energy, and I feel fortunate every time we have a chance to spend time together, as he has become a good friend. Like many others, he has encouraged and supported me on my journey of learning to transcend my pain, frustration, and other blocks to reaching higher states of consciousness.

Processes for Loving Unconditionally

Below are five simple processes to help you open your heart, forgive, release emotional stagnation, and love. While they can be practiced separately if you have time, it is more powerful to do them all together.

Write Your Way to a New Perspective

Write down conditions you place on others in order to love them. For example, what behaviors or actions make you withdraw your love? Do you judge and place labels that limit the love you share with them? What if you could see others from a new perspective? What if you actually saw them as pure, beautiful souls who may have forgotten who they really are and are now trying to find their way in the world, which is full of extremes and contradictions?

Feel the difference in your body as you begin to experience them from a new perspective. In order to have greater compassion, you may need to place yourself in their shoes and see life from their point of view.

Practice Forgiveness

To love yourself and others unconditionally, you need to practice the art of forgiveness. Forgive yourself for your imperfections and forgive others theirs. A simple process you can do is to picture them in front of you as you say silently or out loud:

> *Divine Healing Intelligence, please help me release any feelings of* _____ _____ [insert feelings you have toward this person, which could include victimhood, anger, frustration, resentment, distrust, misunderstanding, hurt, or rejection] *toward* _____ [insert person's name].

Dear _____ [insert person's name], *I forgive you for*
_____ [state what you forgive them for]. [If appropriate
say] *Please forgive me for* _____ [state what you would like them
to forgive you for].

*Divine Love, please sweep through us and cleanse any harmful, negative, or judg-
mental feelings and transform them into understanding, clear communication, deeper
compassion, and unconditional love. Thank you.*

Repeat the word "CLEAR" several times, until you feel lighter

Release Emotions

Sit with your spine straight. Bring your arms to the level of your heart, with your palms
facing your chest. You middle fingers should be touching each other, while your other
fingers point directly at each other and your thumbs point upward. Take slow, deep
breaths, then hold your breath for a few moments. Focus on letting go of any emotional
pain and density as you breathe out. Do this for a few minutes.

Heal with Color

Rub your hands together for about a minute, making sure that you rub your palms and
all your fingers against each other. Then hold your hands between two to four inches
apart. You should feel a tingling sensation. Visualize holding a big pink ball of energy.
Focus on this ball of energy and allow it to intensify. Meditate on filling this ball with
the deepest, most Divine unconditional love. Once you feel a sense of expansion, imagine placing the ball of energy into your heart, and allow your heart to grow and expand
with love.

Meditate on Love

Meditate on love every day. Ask yourself regularly: *Am I experiencing this situation from a perspective of fear or of love? If I was seeing this person or this event from a*

perspective of love, how would I feel? How would I respond to this person? What actions would I take?

Be open to connecting to and spending time with people who emanate the energy of love. The more time you spend with someone who is living life from a perspective of unconditional love, the easier it is for you to evolve and access this state yourself.

Make a commitment to yourself to spend at least five minutes a day for the next three months, meditating on unconditional love and viewing people from a more loving accepting perceptive.

10

HOW YOU CAN RECOGNIZE AND ATTRACT SOUL MATES AND TWIN SOULS

I have heard many people talking about soul mates and twin souls.
I want to understand what a twin soul is, and how is it different from a soul mate?
How can a person recognize when they have met their twin soul?
Is there a way to attract a twin soul or, at least, prepare to meet them?
Also are there other types of soul mates, and if so, what are they?

The subject of soul mates and soul families in the spirit world and in physical reality is a hugely complex one about which much has been written. I am constantly exploring this fascinating topic through my personal experiences, workshops, writing, meditation, and communication with higher guidance. I hope this chapter stimulates your curiosity and compels you on your own journey to discover more.

The romanticized concept of a soul mate—as the ideal lover who, once you meet him or her, completes your life in exactly the way you have fantasized about—has caused many people a lot of suffering. This could be due to so many of us waiting for the "perfect" partner and feeling disappointed when we meet our actual soul mates, as it is very rare (if ever) that they are able to fulfill the projection of what we desire them to be. Since we can share various lifetimes with our soul mates, they can play many different roles, not just that of a lover.

Thus, we must expand our concepts of who soul mates are and the real purpose of these powerful, life altering connections we may be fortunate enough to experience.

Finding Your Soul Mate

Unfortunately, there is no foolproof process that leads you to your twin soul or soul mates. However, the deeper you connect with your own heart to experience your own wholeness, the more likely you are to attract loving, spiritual, evolved beings into your life. When you are open and receptive to your Higher Self and Divine Guidance, you can reconnect with your twin soul without necessarily meeting him or her in the physical world. You may experience a strong link with your twin soul for many years before you meet.

The subject of soul mates is a fascinating one that has given occasion to many ideas and interpretations. Certain people believe soul mates are people who challenge us the most; others believe they should be our perfect lovers; some feel they are parts of us and can come in a variety of forms, sizes, sexes, and ages.

Soul mates can offer incredible support, growth, and opportunities to know ourselves more intimately, open our hearts, and lead fuller lives. And we have several soul mates who come in and out of our lives. At times, we meet and recognize them, and at other times, they pass us by.

In romantic relationships, soul mates make great partners, as they share a lot of mutual understanding and love. Soul mates also feel a deep attraction to each other, and may experience heightened intuition or deep insights about each other. They can often tell when the other is thinking of them, or when something wonderful or challenging has happened to their soul partner.

Soul mates can also be extremely challenging partners, pushing every button we have, and exposing our most secret and unprocessed pain. If they are selfish and unevolved, they can be virtually impossible to live with. We may feel a deep connection with a soul mate and be able to communicate on the soul level, but in a human body, the dynamics can be too explosive and painful.

On the other hand, soul mates can offer essential support, and be loyal friends and important teachers who change the direction and flow of your life. Sometimes they come into your life, make a big splash, and leave. This can inspire a lot of soul-searching and strengthen your spiritual stamina. Although it is challenging to let go of a soul mate relationship in a physical life, it is important to understand that soul connections are eternal. You may have a very clear agreement with a soul mate to separate at a particular moment in your life in order to grow and evolve.

Karmic factors and soul agreements play a huge role in whether or when you meet a soul mate and the nature of the connection.

Soul Groups

From my research and personal experience, I believe that our soul mates are people who come from our soul group in the spirit world. They are souls who travel with us through diverse journeys and challenges, and through a wide variety of lifetimes and experiences, often evolving at a similar pace. Relationships with soul mates are rich and profound, imbedded with a deep sense of knowing, and of loving one another independent of time or distance.

You may already be aware that you have a primary soul family in the spirit world, which is made up of souls who love, support, and look out for each other. Oftentimes, they grow, learn, and explore spiritual and physical life at the same pace. Your primary soul family might have a dozen or fewer members, while your secondary soul group can consist of hundreds or even thousands of souls. Your parents and siblings are usually from one of the affiliated soul groups.

There are certain souls in your secondary soul group with whom you may choose to explore karmic relationships over one or more lifetimes. You can also agree to make short or extensive appearances in each other's lives, and play simple or complex roles. During past life regressions, many people recognize the souls who have traveled with them on various journeys in different bodies.

Types of Soul Mates

On the next few pages, I outline some of the different soul connections to help you recognize the type of soul connection you have with a person. Though there may be an unlimited number of types, I am sharing the ones I (and other people I know personally) have experienced.

Twin Soul

The twin soul, also known as a twin flame or a primary soul mate, is often referred to as one of the closest, deepest, most extraordinary relationships a person can experience. Some people say that a twin soul is one soul that has split in half; others say that a twin flame was the last soul you separated from before you became an individual soul, thus you are always looking for that part of you that was lost. As we have several soul mates, we can experience similar things with more than one person; however, a twin-soul connection is very specific and quite different from other soul connections. I share my extraordinary experience with a twin soul later in this chapter.

Complementary Souls

Complementary souls can, at times, perfectly balance each other. Together, they can be seen as yin and yang. While yin is feminine, soft, and emotional, yang is fiery, strong, and masculine. Though they seem like they are opposing, they are also complementary, assisting each other to continuously expand, grow, and evolve. They interact within a greater whole, and bring out each other's light and shadow. Each one contains the essence of the other, and once they meet, they often feel like they are one person and cannot exist without the other—even though they can.

It is rare for perfectly complementary souls to be on earth at the same time. If they choose to incarnate together, it is often for the purpose of evolution, to bring healing and transformation to our planet.

Complementary souls either uplift and encourage each other, or push each other toward experiencing their greatest unprocessed pain and karma. This can lead to an intensely challenging and profound exploration of the dark night of the soul.

When these souls meet, they feel a deep connection and know that they will rock each other's worlds. The love between them can be so fierce that if they do not communicate clearly and regularly, and find ways to help and support each other through their challenges, they may sabotage their relationship.

A separation from a complementary soul can be hurtful, traumatic, and agonizing, and deep-seated feelings of abandonment, rejection, and neglect can arise.

In this case, the opportunity is for each to find wholeness in himself or herself, create a stronger connection to the Divine Source, and bond when the time is right. This could be at a later stage in the same life, when the complementary souls have grown in wisdom, or when they meet again in the spirit world.

Split Soul

Split souls are a rarity. It is believed that before incarnating in this life or in earlier lives, one soul decided to split into two or more parts in order to lead several lives at once. There are usually two reasons for this: either a soul has done some questionable, often harmful deeds in several lives and has decided that it needs to split to balance out its karma; or the soul is quite evolved and believes that it can make a greater impact and progress faster to higher states of consciousness if it splits. This kind of connection is quite testing, as the people involved often experience similar things at the same time and strongly influence each other, even if they are on opposite sides of the world.

If one person hurts the other, both suffer intensely and can feel like they are scarring each other's hearts. Whatever one does, whether to uplift or to sabotage, impacts the other.

Split souls can experience strong feelings of being inseparable and melting into each other. When together, they can read each other's energy and accurately access what is happening in each other's lives. They can also recall the same past life experiences, as it is really the same soul experiencing other lives. They can also know personal information about challenging experiences that have occurred to each other in this life.

As they feel a deep, unbreakable link, this can cause split souls to push each other's buttons and create large conflicts. If they chose to be born in the same time, they often take on bodies that are quite different from each other and are on opposite sides of the world. Their mission can be to experience opposing sides of life while learning as much as possible. If they meet in this life, they require gentleness, and a deep level of compassion and forgiveness for themselves and each other, particularly at the start, as it can be a very dramatic and confusing experience.

My Story: Split Soul

While I was not familiar with a split soul experience until I met Fred, I have since encountered several people who have connected with a split soul in this life. Like other soul mates, split-soul connections can choose to experience a romantic relationship, often to heal feelings of separation from one another, and to experience the oneness of the female and male polarities. However, split soul relationships can also be with a parent, sibling, child, friend, or someone else close to you.

My split-soul experience was completely unexpected. When I met Fred, I instantly saw his soul. His energy was magnetic. I couldn't help being drawn to him and vice versa. When he saw me, he told me that he witnessed a past life we had experienced. This was the first time he had ever seen a past life.

We did a heart connection process together, which required each of us to hold the energy of the other person's heart. When Fred held mine, I felt like a huge, missing soul fragment came back into my body and soul, and I could not stop crying. It was as if the shell that was encasing my heart was melting, and I felt an incredible sense of expansion.

When I asked him what he had done, he explained that he had brought both of our hearts together, and they became one full heart. The only other time I had this experience was with my twin soul, Piotr, and I had never told Fred about this. (I tell this story on page 134.)

Besides this, we have had numerous synchronistic occurrences and visions to clarify our connection. Incredibly, Fred was able to recall several of my most challenging experiences in this life and obtain detailed information that he could not have possibly known. We have also felt many things at the same time, including having pain in the same part of our bodies, simultaneously discovering strange information about a place we had never discussed, receiving identical spiritual insights, appearing in front of each other in an energetic form, and sending energy and healing to each other when we needed it without being asked.

When I asked Fred what a split-soul connection meant to him, he said, "I believe that this rare meeting is so powerful that it can instantly raise your level of evolution and bring you to a higher state of consciousness, the next level your soul is meant to go to."

Due to our varied life experiences and belief systems our relationship was tumultuous at the beginning. However, we now support each other in a loving and gentle manner.

It is also important to note that while we are aware of the depth the connection we feel, we are not overly concerned with labels but more with the experience of evolving and supporting each other. Everyone has their own unique experience, so please honor yourself and be gentle, especially if your soul mate does not yet understand the complexity and beauty of your connection.

How to Recognize a Soul Mate Connection

There is a familiarity and a powerful connection between you. You may feel like you have known each other forever.

It is likely that you have met through an unexpected or unusual set of circumstances.

Often, there are obstacles that may prevent you from being together; this could be from living in other places, having a partner, not having the same sexual preferences, being born in different cultures, having differing religious circumstances, and so forth.

When you are connected with this person, everything in life feels heightened, purer, clearer, bigger, and more profound.

The relationship is deeply loving and devotional; you are happy to go out of your way to support him or her and vice versa. You would do things for this person that you would usually never dream of doing for others.

You help melt each other's resistance to love and open each other's hearts, often touching parts of yourselves that have been frozen or feel raw.

When you are together, extraordinary things and synchronicities happen regularly.

You can read each other's thoughts and often feel what is happening in the other person's life.

You are mirrors for each, experiencing similar or identical life circumstances and events at or near the same timeframe.

You trust this person, and feel like you can pour out your heart and share your deepest thoughts and secrets.

The more time you spend together, the more you grow, expand, and become wiser.

You give to each other from the most loving and tender place in your heart without the need to be repaid in any way, because you really want to. Giving is joyful.

You help each other see and transcend flaws and weaknesses, which assists you to grow and gain wisdom.

When you meet, you may receive flashes of each other's past lives.

If the connection is meant to lead to a life partnership, you may receive a message that you are meant to be together.

You may have dreams or visions about a soul mate before you meet him or her.

The Challenging Aspects of Soul Mate Relationships

Sometimes, the souls that are closest to you can choose to play people who greatly test you, while helping you heal and resolve difficult karmic patterns. The challenge is to see a bigger picture, and recognize that they are not here to hurt you but to help you—help you to become more courageous, forgiving, loving, healthy, strong, creative, flexible, intuitive, and refined, among many other qualities.

As you awaken and remember who you really are, you begin to focus more on your soul's journey and less on the everyday nitty-gritty of life. Having said that, it is important to live a grounded, practical, responsible life. For instance, if you meet a soul mate whom you desire to have a romantic relationship with but one of you is not ready or available in an emotional, mental, or physical manner, I would encourage you to acknowledge to yourself (and possibly your soul mate, if it is appropriate) that you would love to share your life with them, but because of the circumstances, this is not possible. Try to find a way this person can be in your life in a healing manner, where you help each other without creating destruction.

It is important to understand that you have a contract with your soul mate to play different roles in each other's lives. Although you are unlikely to miss a soul mate you have an agreement with, it is possible to resist, avoid, and push them out of your life, as you still have free choice on the human level. Fear can strongly influence your decisions and behavior.

I have watched countless people make the most loving soul connections only to pass on a chance to really get to know each other, because of earthly fears, judgments, laziness, jealousy, misunderstandings, selfishness, and self-sabotaging tendencies.

Intensely protecting your heart, being pessimistic, and not allowing anyone to come close to you can repel even the most persistent soul mate.

All soul mates will initiate profound transformation, love, and at times, a sense of deep discomfort inside you. Perhaps true evolution occurs on the cusp of chaos and order. As you deal with one challenging situation and breathe a sigh of relief, life provides you with the next opportunity to learn, grow, develop, and master the skills you require to go to the next level of consciousness and enlightenment.

Soul Connections in Our Past Lives and Between Lives

I remember having an incredible session that showed me what occurs to our souls in past lives and in between lives. During this session, I was taken into a significant past life with an important soul mate, who was my brother in that life. Our parents had died, and we were trying to survive on our own. My brother made a vow to look after me. However, when I was about thirteen, I got the news of his death. I was completely devastated. Even during the regression, I cried uncontrollably, and my heart felt like it was being torn into pieces. That life deeply resonated with me, and I felt like it was stored in my soul and cellular memories.

In that lifetime, after my brother died, I became interested in natural medicine and shamanism. I learned about the healing properties of nature and eventually became a valued leader in the community.

My ability to communicate with nature, spirits, and the Divine was highly developed in that life. And when I died, it was through conscious choice. During a beautiful ceremony, I observed as my soul floated out of my body and was immediately met by my soul mate.

It was interesting to see that, although I was a fairly wise leader in that life, my first question to my soul mate was, "Why did you leave me?" He answered that he had stayed until he felt I was strong and courageous enough to follow my soul's path. He told me that had he remained longer, I would not have taken the path of becoming a spiritual guide for many people. He shared that it was an agreement we made before we entered that life. I felt healed and complete after hearing and understanding his reasons for leaving.

Being able to explore our past lives and the spans between our lives can help us understand our soul agreements, forgive, move on, and heal our fear of loss and death.

My Story: Finding My Twin Soul

I can only truly talk about a twin soul from my own experience. I met mine on my second teaching trip in Paris. It was both a trying and an extraordinary time. I arrived a few days before the national French presidential election, and everyone I met in Paris seemed permeated with fear. Within hours of landing on French soil, I found out that I had no accommodation. My organizer, who was also my translator, had an emotional crisis and told me that she was no longer able to work with me; and the one person I knew who spoke English was out of the country. I felt ready to pack my bags and go home.

However, I knew that even though I wanted to run, I needed to understand why I was drawn so strongly to Paris. The answer arrived a few days later while I was sitting in a taxi. I was looking out the window, taking in the little cobblestone streets and contemplating *What am I doing in Paris?* when I saw a massive sign in English that read "Be Love." I knew then that I had come to Paris to learn and teach the real meaning of love. The moment I embraced this intention, incredible things began to occur. I was offered a place to stay, I found a new organizer, my conferences were full, and my workshops sold out.

It was also in Paris that I found my twin soul, Piotr, whom I met at his couture boutique. (I share more about my first meeting with Piotr in chapter 17, "How You Can Clear Your Space and House.") For now, it is enough to say that our first meeting was incredible, inevitable, and without a doubt, Divinely inspired. Astonishingly, no matter how I resisted, it was impossible for me not to connect with him.

Although initially Piotr seemed uncomfortable with the idea of healing, within a few hours of meeting me, he asked me for a space clearing and a healing session, and I agreed to do it the following day. During the healing session, I had a phenomenal experience: while Piotr was relaxing on the massage table, I tuned in to his body and was drawn to his heart.

I then saw a vision in which his heart came out of his chest and connected to my heart. Then his heart kissed mine and I heard "Thank you." The experience was so impactful that I began to feel dizzy and disoriented. Powerful surges of energy moved through my whole being. It felt as if a deep, ancient part of my heart was awakening.

Although I had done thousands of healing sessions, I had never felt anything like it. The experience definitely captured my interest.

The connection between Piotr and me was extraordinary. Ever since I was six, I had experienced an odd feeling that I had a brother with light hair and blue eyes who was three years older. As a young boy, Piotr fit this description perfectly. When I first saw him, I felt like his image was deeply familiar—as if it was etched in my soul. For two years before we met, I had the most vivid dreams about a blond, European man with blue eyes. Piotr told me that a few months before we met, he had a strong feeling that he would meet someone who would change his life; when we met, he recognized that I was the person he had been waiting for. Within days of meeting, we felt like we had known each other forever. Although Piotr had little interest in spirituality before we met, he devoured every bit of information I shared with him. What impressed me most was his natural ability to swiftly grasp the healing work I was teaching.

Less than a week later, Piotr told me he could accurately tap in to my world and read my mind, know my feelings, and sense what I was experiencing, whether I was asleep or awake. And I could do the same with him. We were even able to send each other telepathic messages when we needed the other's help or wanted to catch up.

Both Piotr and I were in committed relationships, and neither of us knew how to interpret and deal with the feelings of deep soul love we were experiencing toward each other. This love did not feel romantic but was more spiritual and Divine. One evening, while having dinner with Piotr, I had a persistent thought in my head: *Twin soul, twin soul, twin soul.* As I had no idea what a twin soul was, I found this thought quite disturbing.

When I returned to Australia and shared my experience with Paul, he helped me to find out more about what a twin soul is.

Since I am not the strongest believer in labels, I would not have categorized my relationship with Piotr as a twin soul had I not heard the words repeated in my head over and over again. As I was completely overwhelmed and confused by our connection, being able to read about what a twin soul is has helped me to put our relationship into perspective and handle some of the more challenging aspects of our connection.

Meeting Piotr rocked and transformed my whole world, just as meeting me changed his. When I asked Piotr to share how he felt when we met, he said,

"I experienced a feeling of happiness and safety like I had never felt before. I also had a strong knowing that I had met a part of myself that had been missing for a long time. It was a relief, like finally I'm whole and from now on, we know we'll always be there for each other.

"I can now relax and unconsciously stop searching."

Although my relationship with Paul went through some challenges after I met Piotr, I instinctively felt that it would deepen my love and connection with Paul. From meeting Piotr, I have learned what true devotion, unconditional love, and Divine connection really is. All I know is that when you meet your twin soul and have the opportunity to get to know them, you truly experience Divinity, and touch the essence of who you are as a soul.

Meeting your twin soul is not necessarily an easy ride. In fact, it can be the most challenging, painful, and difficult experience of your life. Just as your twin soul can make you feel the most heightened state of bliss and melt your heart, he or she can also take you to the deepest pain, hurt, rejection, and anger you may ever experience. In other words, they really make you grow.

If you are experiencing the challenging side of a twin-soul relationship, I encourage you to not cut and run. Instead, be gentle, take some time to calm down, and become aware of what your twin soul is bringing up for you to face. Then work on your own issues before you reconnect.

I have heard many stories from my workshop participants about meeting their twin souls. Some met in foreign countries, some were in other relationships, some were much older or much younger, some were best friends, and others were siblings. Very few were lovers. After reflecting on this for a while, I realized that if twin souls are extremely similar, it would make sense that, as souls, they would choose other people to help them grow, expand, and experience intimate relationships. It would not work for them to be a couple in every life or to spend all their time together, as they would not grow and learn from interacting with diversity of people.

Letting Go: When Soul Mates Must Take Different Paths

Sometimes, you will spend multiple years with a soul mate, believing that you are destined to be together forever, only to discover that, at a particular moment, both of you feel that you want to move in different directions.

One of the most touching interviews I have conducted was with Richard Bach, the author of many bestselling books, including *Jonathan Livingston Seagull* and *Illusions*. Richard shared that, at one point in his life, he thought soul mates were "two people who have chosen to share a lifetime, and that they would be teachers, one to the other, all through that lifetime. And then they would reflect upon it after that lifetime was finished." He further confided, "I think this belief is true for a lot of people. I thought it was true for me and wrote about it. Then it turned out that Lesley Parish and I had different paths to walk. So that experience, that relationship, that marriage ended, and I understood the idea of a school—that we can have a teacher from whom we can learn an enormous amount, but there is a time when we graduate from that class."[15]

At times, it is healthier (although emotionally painful) to let go of a soul mate who has chosen a different direction from yours. For instance, you may be working on your emotional and spiritual evolution, while he or she feels inclined to drink, take drugs, abuse their body, and sabotage their life.

Even though you may be physically apart, the spiritual link can never be broken, so I suggest that you still connect to and communicate solely with their soul. Visualize this person and talk to their soul, expressing what you need to share. Know that, on some level, you are heard. If it is for your highest good, you will reconnect again in this lifetime, at a more appropriate time.

Making Time for Soul Connections

Beyond my experiences with Piotr and Fred, I have had a number of other soul connections. Most of these were instantly recognizable, and were permeated with feelings of love, familiarity, and warmth. Each time I meet a person with whom I have a soul connection, I feel like I have been invited to the biggest party on earth. I feel deeply grateful to know that I am not alone, and that there are many amazing souls walking the earth that I am here to share my life with.

In my personal life, whenever I meet anyone I feel a soul connection with, I do my best to make time for them, no matter how busy I am. This is because I know that people who are part of our soul group have deep and profound gifts that can help us to raise our vibration, experience incredible states of consciousness, give us courage to follow our dreams, and open our hearts.

Process for Connecting with a Soul Mate or Twin Soul

Even if you have already met your soul mate or twin soul, do this process with them. Feel free to adjust the process to sharing love with them in the now. You may prefer to connect to a soul mate instead of a twin soul, so please adjust anything necessary in this process to suit yourself. (Even though this process is broken up into five sections, you must do all of them together in order to gain the most benefit.)

Create a Clear Intention

First, create a clear intention for connecting with your twin soul. Place your hands on your heart, and focus on opening your heart to your twin soul. You may imagine the doors of your heart opening to welcome your twin soul.

Take some slow deep breaths while focusing on your heart and soul energy.

Imagine that a powerful, golden ray of light enters through your crown chakra and moves into your third eye, amplifying your intention to connect with this much-loved soul. Soul mates can often receive telepathic messages from each other and feel drawn to connect.

Take a few more deep breaths, and then visualize the gold ray of light moving toward your throat.

Say the following statement, adding anything else you feel inspired to add: "I allow the Divine Love from my heart and soul to now flow toward the heart and soul of my twin soul, and to surround them with love, tenderness, gentleness, compassion, and warmth. I ask that any hardships or challenges my twin soul may be experiencing be softened and resolved with ease and grace. If it is for the highest good of all, I ask that our paths meet in the physical world, and that we recognize and support each other's journey through life with our hearts and souls.

If we are not to meet in this physical world, then I ask that we experience a deeply satisfying spiritual connection and assist each other. I also ask that any soul mates or beings who can assist me to grow will now be directed toward me—beings who can awaken the love, passion, and sweetness in my heart, and bring me joy and uplift me. Please give me clear and recognizable signs when a twin soul or a soul mate is in my vicinity. I am now ready to receive them with open arms and an open heart! Thank you, Divine Spirit."

Repeat the word "CLEAR" several times, until you feel lighter.

Feel the intensity of what you have just invoked.

Share Love with Your Soul Mate

Imagine that the soul of your twin or a soul mate is now standing in front of you, emanating love, bliss, and delight at simply being close to you. Take in the sweetness of this connection.

Allow the golden ray of light to move toward your heart and envelop it. Relax and soften, and allow yourself to savor the sensation. Imagine that there is an energy cord between your heart and your twin soul's heart. Through this cord, send your soul mate as much love, tenderness, and warmth as you can muster. Then sense the care, appreciation, and affection they return to you. Observe this exquisite energy circulating between you and your twin soul.

Purify Your Heart

Let the love, warmth, and kindness from your twin soul purify your heart and wash away any pain, disappointment, or rejection you may have experienced in your relationships with others. Replace the hurt with gratitude for your life, and open yourself to the possibility of reconnecting with one or more soul mates at the perfect time and in the perfect way, so that together you can explore the depth of unimaginable and eternal love. Allow this love to move through your whole body and energy field, releasing and cleansing any fear or resistance into the earth beneath you, which can transmute all negativity and surround you with a soft, nurturing energy.

Become Grounded with the Energy of Love

Ask that this process be done with ease and grace. When you feel that the process is complete, move your body gently, focusing on grounding this energy of love into your feet. The more grounded and connected you are to your heart and to the earth's loving vibration, the faster amazing experiences and loving people will come into your life.

Although this process is soft and gentle, it is very powerful, so I encourage everyone to practice it.

love. Allow this love to move through your whole body and energy field, releasing and cleansing any fear or resistance into the earth beneath you, which can transmute all negativity and surround you with a soft, morning energy.

Become Grounded with the Energy of Love

Ask that this process be done with ease and grace. When you feel that the process is complete, move our body gently, focusing on grounding this energy of love into your feet. The more grounded and connected you are to your heart and to the earth's loving vibration, the faster amazing experiences and loving people will come into your life. Although this process is soft and gentle, it is very powerful, so I encourage everyone to practice it.

11

HOW YOU CAN DISCOVER AND HEAL PAST LIVES

What is your view of past lives and how they affect us?
Can you give some examples of how understanding past lives can be helpful?

Through my many years of exploring and researching health, wellness, spirituality, and metaphysics, I have learned that we are complex, spiritual beings who have had many different incarnations and experiences. Since the world is going through a great awakening, more and more people are discovering the benefits of learning from their past lives and hastening their evolution. They feel that it is unnecessary to repeat the same mistakes over and over if there is an opportunity to do things in an easier way—through healing, forgiving, and learning from the past.

Learning Lessons from Our Past Lives

Each life, a soul leaves its marks, experiences, impressions, and karmic patterns, which need to be resolved. Thus, it is common to have themes repeated in several lifetimes, until the soul feels that it has satisfactorily understood the important lesson.

The physical world is a place of great contrast, which gives a soul the opportunity to grow and evolve. If a soul did not manage to learn, heal, experience, or fulfill its intention in one life, then it might desire or be encouraged by its guides to return and try again.

When a soul chooses to enter a new life, it usually does so enthusiastically, with the understanding and anticipation of what will be experienced. The soul knows that this is an opportunity to expand, learn, develop, and make new choices. It brings invisible records (the Akashic Records) of all the relevant past experiences it needs to work on. Stored in the soul's chakras and vibrational field, these records set up powerful patterns, which attract the people and experiences it intends to encounter.

These experiences are not necessarily hard or challenging; in fact, they can be extraordinary, awakening, loving, and deeply uplifting. The Akashic Records also hold all the gifts, abilities, and talents a soul has acquired from previous incarnations.

A soul who has had many experiences of being a follower may decide to rise up, become a leader, and go through the steps of transforming past beliefs and limitations to do so. Sometimes this will be done with a conscious awareness of the existence of past lives; at other times, it will occur naturally, without the need to revisit and learn from the past.

I have discovered that once a person understands where their patterns, pain, or a difficult experience is coming from, and lets it go on the vibrational, emotional, and mental levels, their physical reality changes dramatically. He or she may experience an amazing physical healing, release a haunting emotional pattern, improve a difficult relationship, feel lighter and more empowered, decide to pursue their abandoned dreams, and feel more at ease with life.

I have witnessed and experienced many past-life regressions. Some of these experiences gave vital clues to the lessons that needed to be learned, making a huge difference in my life and other people's lives. Most past-life regressions transform participants' points of view and result in wiser, more loving and forgiving people. Some past lives may give you insights into what it is like to have beautiful, peaceful, intuitive relationships; others may demonstrate the pain of loss, betrayal, separation, and heartbreak.

In my own experiences, I saw lives where I took charge, became a leader, and made both excellent and poor decisions that cost me my life as well as the lives of people close to me. The discovery has been fascinating, making me understand my talents, abilities, and weaknesses in a deeper and more profound way.

This exploration has also made me appreciate several of my family members, as I see them from a new point of view. It's important to note that we often return with souls we feel a connection with.

Helen's Story: A Mother and Son Reconnected

Helen was at her wit's end when she came to me for help. She was having difficulty connecting with Andrew, her three-year-old, who constantly threw tantrums, shouted, screamed, and kicked her.

I discovered that Helen went through a very tough time before her pregnancy and did not want a second child. When I tuned in to Helen's energy, I saw a dark cord attached from her womb to Andrew, and the cord was heavy, full of negative beliefs, such as Helen not wanting her son. To Andrew, these beliefs felt poisonous, and he rebelled against them by throwing tantrums. I was shown that Helen needed to make a decision about whether she did or did not want him. When Helen heard this, she began to cry uncontrollably.

I was also shown that, in another life, Helen and Andrew were a couple, and Andrew had been dragged away to a war and killed. Helen was heartbroken. In this life, she felt fearful of loving Andrew because she could not handle the idea of being separated from him. I helped Helen clear the cord between Andrew and her, worked on her energy centers, and brought back soul fragments of love and trust.

Helen shared with me that after the healing session, Andrew woke, called her to him, kissed her all over her face, and said, "Mummy, I love you." She told me that whenever she looks at him, she melts. It seemed like their relationship transformed overnight.

Sometimes, seeing a particular past life can help you change your perspectives about important events and heal close relationships.

Taking Responsibility for Our Past and Future Lives

Karmic patterns often determine what kind of lessons we have come to learn and whether we experience our lives through ease or hardship. The law of karma requires that everything comes full cycle; any good or harm we have done will return to us—the universal law of cause and effect. Exploring past lives can help people take responsibility in the present and give them the impetus to work on a particular challenge. If a person knows that they cannot avoid or run away from a problem, even through dying, the motivation to resolve it increases.

Recently, I spoke with some people about the importance of looking after our environment. After listening to them, I realized that although some were concerned about the state of the planet because of their children, many only cared about how things were going to work for the next thirty to fifty years, until the end of their lives. None seemed to consider the idea that they might return here, and that it would be worth looking after the planet so that they had something positive to return to. When I mentioned this factor, a new discussion arose about taking responsibility for our future.

Sebastian's Story: Amazing Physical Healing

I met Sebastian when he was thirteen years old. Lisa, Sebastian's mother, saw me on television and called me to book a healing session, feeling like there was new hope for her son after years of searching for a cure for his juvenile arthritis. The disease had affected his right knee and foot, which were both extremely swollen. He was constantly in pain and, at times, needed crutches.

Sebastian was young and positive, so it did not seem that his problem came from negative beliefs or feelings that he was harboring in this life. He was experiencing typical younger-brother syndrome with his older brother but otherwise was quite confident and sure of himself.

I taught Sebastian several processes to release pain from his legs and to improve his relationship with his brother. Within a short time, Sebastian was free of pain and crutches. However, the swelling did not seem to budge. Then Sebastian came to a workshop where I taught about past lives. After

146

experiencing a past-life regression, Sebastian, who was usually very casual and calm, became extremely emotional while holding his swollen knee.

After Sebastian calmed down, he shared his experience. He saw himself with his mother in a past life, but in that life, his mother was his older sister. He had a vision of them swimming together in the ocean without noticing a shark nearby. Sebastian cried out when he realized that the shark had attacked him and bit off his right leg, just above his knee. His sister, blaming herself, was so distraught that she vowed to look after him forever. Due to this trauma, Sebastian has since brought his arthritis into each life. In his current life, he and his mother came together as an opportunity to transcend and heal the past, and to support each other to realize their dreams.

I asked both Sebastian and Lisa to do a forgiveness process together and to give each other permission to live their dreams. Sebastian's dream was to become a professional golfer, and Lisa's was to become more healthy and happy, relocate, travel, and bring more creativity into her life.

Interestingly, within a few weeks of past-life healing, Sebastian's swelling completely disappeared. He began taking his golf practice seriously and has won many trophies since. Lisa began to focus on herself, has become more confident, started traveling, has manifested a new home, and is exploring her other dreams.

Pascal and Angelica's Story: Reclaiming Intuitive Abilities

Another incredible experience occurred when I was teaching a workshop in Europe. Pascal and Angelica, two of the participants, seemed extremely uncomfortable with each other. They constantly and teased one another—to the point that I had to intervene and separate them.

Both complained about their difficulty in tuning in and seeing things. So it blew us all away when, after I'd guided everyone through a past-life regression process, Pascal and Angelica shared almost identical accounts of being together in a previous life.

They had been lovers, and Angelica was gifted with intuitive abilities. She would just know things about the people she met, and she received messages and predictions about their future. Pascal was an explorer who sailed the seas and discovered new territories. Before Pascal's last journey, Angelica felt that his life could be in danger. Although she usually shared her premonitions, she refused to believe that something could happen to the man she was supposed to marry, and decided to ignore her intuition.

Pascal was completely in love with Angelica and felt that she was the love of his life. When Pascal left on his trip, he came across some danger that almost killed him, and he was lost at sea for a long time. Angelica was informed that he had died, and she blamed herself harshly. In her distraught state, she disconnected from her intuitive abilities and had no idea that Pascal was still alive and searching for her. She married another man, and when Pascal found her, he felt completely betrayed and broken-hearted. He vowed to never allow himself to trust another woman or to be with a woman he loved, because it hurt so much to see her with another man.

Incredibly, both Pascal and Angelica cried while retelling their story. Even more astonishing, they knew each other's past-life names and told their stories from their unique points of view.

In her present life, Angelica had deeply desired to tap in to her intuitive abilities, without success. She also felt that she was undeserving of a great relationship with a man. Pascal always picked women he did not love, for fear of being betrayed and abandoned.

I led Angelica and Pascal through a process of deep forgiveness and healing. Initially, Angelica was so emotional that she could not speak, so I asked her to communicate to Pascal with her soul. Pascal looked deep into Angelica's eyes, and saw the profound pain and shame she was carrying. He helped her forgive this old wound and feel safe in trusting her intuition, and reconnecting her with higher intelligence.

As this amazing communication across lives was occurring, the energy in the room was absolutely electric. We were witnessing a miracle healing. After the process was complete, everyone commented that both Pascal and Angelica looked younger, lighter, and more alive.

Pascal told me that he felt he had finally understood the reasons for his destructive behavior. He also said his depression had disappeared, and he felt a lot happier. He gave me a big hug and thanked me for helping him come back to life. As for Angelica, she was able to reclaim her confidence, intuition, and creativity. She also stopped blaming herself and became more open to finding a satisfying, loving relationship. Both went into their lives feeling cleansed and renewed, with the intention to make new choices.

Go to this link to read more transformational stories related to past-life healing.
http://innasegal.com/the-secret-of-life-wellness-downloads/transformational-stories

Sharing Past Lives

I have had countless people come up to me after workshops, interviews, talks, and healing sessions to tell me that they have a strong connection with me, assuring me that we've had many past lives together. I believe that exploring past lives is a sacred and personal experience for understanding and healing your life. And sharing about your past lives with others should be done in a receptive and respectful environment.

In all the years that I have taught past life regression, there has been only a handful of people with whom I truly felt that we had a connection that went across time and space. Usually, our recognition has been instant, deep, and unusual, often accompanied by strong feelings of love and care, as well as a many synchronicities.

In most of these cases, both of us were aware of the profound connection we were experiencing. There have also been a few times when I've had negative reactions to people for no apparent reason. In my own exploration, I discovered that I had shared some past lives with them, and we needed to rebalance our karma. Upon releasing the charge and transforming the traumas in our past lives, our relationships became neutral. Often, they departed from my life in a peaceful way.

Past-life regression can offer many glimpses and understandings into our complex and mysterious life experiences. But be aware that not every connection you feel is related to a past life. Before you share your past-life experience with another person, make sure that person is ready and receptive to hear something like this, and that you don't scare or alienate them.

Though I believe that exploring past lives can be extremely valuable, I encourage you to primarily focus on your present life to improve your current situation. Work with your past lives to gain more compassion and to heal, as the stories in this chapter demonstrate.

Process for Dissolving Past-Life Karma

You can do this process as part of the past-life healing process or on its own, when you feel ready to release karma with a person or situation. You can also use it in conjunction with the cord-clearing process on page 188. Think about a situation or a person that you feel has created karma in your life when you repeat the following statement.

Say: "Divine Source, please help me evolve and embrace the light. I vow to do my absolute best to undo any wrongs I have done and heal any wounds I have caused. I now choose to perform all my actions for the highest good of all and to follow my Divine Guidance. Thank you."

Repeat the word "CLEAR" several times, until you feel lighter.

Go to this link to work with an audio recording where I guide you through the past-life healing process described below.
https://soundcloud.com/beyond-words-publishing/inna-segal-past-life

Process for Past-Life Healing

If you are new to past-life healing, it is advisable to use a past-life regression practitioner or a hypnotherapist to guide you through your past-life healing. If you are familiar with this type of work and feel comfortable trying it on your own, you can use the process below or listen to an audio recording I have made. You may also like to ask a friend or a family member to read the process to you if you are reading it in a language other than English.

This process will guide you back through your life to the time before you were born. Please allow yourself to be as open as possible. It is normal to experience doubts or feel like you are making things up. Persevere, however, as the information you receive could be extremely important and help you heal. Sometimes the clarity will come later, so write down your experiences and store them somewhere safe, so that you can refer to them in the future.

Relax

Give yourself between thirty to forty minutes of uninterrupted time. Sit or lie down, and make yourself comfortable. Breathe deeply; allow your body to soften and relax. Let go of any tension, worries, or daily concerns, and focus on slowing down and unwinding. Allow the intelligence of your body to help you dissolve any stress until your body feels soft and relaxed.

Set an Intention

Intend that your Divine Wisdom will support you on this journey, and take you to a deeper awareness of yourself and your past experiences.

Connect with a Spiritual Guide

Focus on your life. Imagine yourself becoming light. Ask that a spiritual guide assist you with this journey. This guide may show up in the form of your best friend, a relative, or a spiritual teacher. The most important thing is to feel safe and supported.

Go Back in Time

Picture taking your guide's hand and floating back in time. Observe the last ten years of your life drift by. Then move further and further back until you see yourself as a child.

Now go even further back, to when you were a baby. Don't worry if you can't remember or see clearly; just allow your consciousness to move back in time until you experience yourself as a soul before you merged with your body.

Feel the lightness, freedom, and expansion of being a soul. Let yourself play and rejoice for a few moments, or just rest in the silence and peacefulness. Then imagine that your guide is leading you toward a beautiful green-and-purple light.

You float toward the light and notice a doorway. Your guide encourages you to enter the room. Once you come into the room, you become aware that it is full of mirrors. Each mirror shows a life you have previously experienced. Allow yourself to be drawn to a mirror that can give you a deeper insight into whatever is occurring in this life that you need to heal or transform. When you see or sense the mirror, allow your guide to support you while you move through this mirror into a life that you have already lived. Imagine literally walking through the mirror and into a new environment.

Ask Questions

Once you have arrived into this life, begin to look around and ask questions. You may receive intuitive insights, images, or feelings, or be shown the events you are inquiring about. Don't be concerned if the messages don't come instantly; just be patient and gentle with yourself. Allow yourself to become aware of who you are in that life.

Are you male or female?

How old are you?

Where are you?

What year is it?

What is happening around you?

What are you feeling?

Be patient with yourself and open to receiving the appropriate answers.

Experience Powerful Moments

Allow your guide to take you to the most important or most powerful moments in your life. Sense and observe what happened. At times, you may feel very strong emotions in your body. If you do, just allow yourself to feel these and let them go, as they may be stuck in your cellular memories. You can also ask to be given an understanding of what you are feeling and what memories those feelings relate to. If you are just receiving images, ask for as much detail as possible. If the images are too fast, ask them to slow down. This is your experience, and you can direct it.

Become aware of the actions you took in that life: were they positive, loving, and inspiring; or did you behave selfishly, violently, and thoughtlessly? What caused you to act the way you did? Become aware of the people who are in that life with you: Do any seem familiar? Could they also be in your present life? Can you recognize them?

Learn Lessons

Ask your Divine Intelligence what lessons you were trying to learn in that life? Did you learn them? Is there anyone that you need to forgive or be forgiven by? If you are open to this, forgive these people, or ask for forgiveness. Do you need to forgive yourself?

Visualize Change

If that life was difficult, challenging, or traumatic, and you could do things differently, how would you rewrite it? Visualize making more empowering decisions, and observe the ways in which your life would change. Often, profound healing can occur from us learning our lessons and choosing again. Even though you are in a new life, you can still transform the negative energy from your previous lives.

Say a Clearing Statement

Say: "I ask Divine Healing Intelligence to move through my body, releasing, clearing, and healing any pain, struggle, fear, grief, guilt, and self-sabotage that I have brought from this previous life into my current life. I ask that white-and-silver rays of purification pour through my body, cleansing, purifying, and revitalizing my energy systems and emotions to peace, clarity, and wellness. Thank you."

Repeat the word "CLEAR" several times, until you feel lighter.

Take slow, deep breaths, allowing the rays of white-and-silver light to flow through your body.

Ask for Messages

When you feel lighter and more peaceful, ask if there are any messages that are relevant in your present life based on what has occurred in your past life. Allow these messages to come to you. If you do not receive them instantly, know that, at some point in the future, you will be shown what you need to know.

Come Back to the Present

When you feel ready, let your guide take your hand and slowly lead you back to the present. Come back into your body and integrate your new experience. This time you'll see that you made a choice to come into this reality to learn, grow, and heal, and that you are a Divine Being who is lovable and worthy of great things.

As you return to the present, breathe slowly and deeply, and allow your body to awaken. You may like to tighten your body for a few seconds and then relax. Tap your feet on the ground to feel more grounded, or simply stretch. Make sure that you take it easy, drink a lot of water, and are gentle with yourself.

12

HOW YOU CAN DISCOVER
YOUR SOUL PURPOSE

Does everyone have a soul purpose?
How would a person go about finding their soul purpose?

Everyone on the physical plane has a soul purpose. A soul is a spiritual entity that is eternal, wise, and ever-evolving. While still in the spirit world, your soul, in conjunction with your guides and wise elders, determines what it needs to learn, understand, and live in the contrasting atmosphere of a physical reality. One aspect of this exploration is karmic; another is stretching past limits to advance spiritually, emotionally, and mentally.

On the soul level, you can only learn and evolve through your own experience. Therefore, the most important thing you can do in life is ask questions and listen to your soul's wisdom.

What Is Your Soul Purpose?

Each person's purpose is to know who they truly are through the experience of exploration and expansion. To discover your soul purpose, you need to become an explorer of your body, consciousness, energy, emotions, spirituality, and life experiences.

By focusing your attention within, sitting quietly, meditating, and breathing consciously, you can become aware of different feelings and sensations that are being stirred in your body. These feelings and sensations are your guidance system. Negative feelings create unpleasant and painful sensations, which show you that the direction you are moving in is limiting, constricting, and hard. When you become aware of feelings of stuckness, you have an opportunity to explore, find another direction, and experience expansion. Thus, when you are connected to yourself, everything guides you toward where your spirit desires to go.

Although I believe that we need to live in a practical, down-to-earth way, I also know that nothing is impossible to a soul following its destiny. Throughout this book, I have shared some of the incredible stories that have occurred in my life and in other people's to demonstrate that we all have a purpose and guidance, if we are receptive.

Your guides and angels may rarely show up in front of you but can communicate with you through a variety of signs. Sometimes you may experience a familiar feeling, or be led to a person, book, class, or place that helps you move forward.

Your soul purpose could include a combination of experiences that your mind does not understand but that your soul needs to learn and grow. Some of these experiences will be extremely enjoyable and heightened; you may even consider them to be peak experiences. Others will be challenging and make you struggle, but through them, you will build your emotional and spiritual stamina.

Your Soul Is Here to Learn

In the spirit world, you enjoy a constant experience of peace, love, and a Divine point of view, but you don't have much of an opportunity to learn and grow firsthand. Thus, learning in the spirit world could be compared to learning in a classroom: someone can tell you that a great chocolate bar can take you to heaven with its delicious cacao, honey, caramel, hazelnuts, and creamy, sweet, nutty texture—and you might salivate at the thought—but until you actually taste it, it will remain a concept.

For most people, birth on the physical plane equals the amnesia of their spiritual heritage. However, the soul still has a strong agenda to fulfill its purpose. Unlike the physical realm, where the idea of your life purpose is connected to a job description, in the spirit world souls see their life purpose as a practical experience where they learn the true meaning of love, compassion, courage, healing, transformation, and creativity.

Through the challenge of dealing with family members, everyday problems, illnesses, difficult relationships, loved ones' deaths, financial struggles, natural disasters, and other traumatic events, we have an opportunity to become more resilient, compassionate, loving, forgiving, creative, innovative, and inspiring.

A soul whose purpose is to become empowered may choose to be born into a family who views their lives from a victim perspective and may cause the new member to feel disempowered. It is this soul's opportunity to become a strong, courageous, compassionate, and inspiring human being while growing up in an opposing environment.

Physical Defects as Blessings

Often, a soul is presented with a selection of several bodies for the optimal fulfillment of its soul purpose. The options can involve healthy or imperfect bodies. It is important to understand that when a soul picks a body, the body is attached to a set of parents with specific points of view on life. Thus, by making a choice of a particular body, the soul takes into consideration the people it will be surrounded by and the challenges it will have to face.

Occasionally, a soul will pick an imperfect body because the learning and the contribution to others can be profound, effective, and far reaching.

I recently read an inspirational story about Lesley, a young woman who was born without any arms. Lesley can write, drive, talk on the phone, type, and fly a plane.

Stuart was born with no arms and one small foot with two toes. Despite this, he surfs, swims, and plays golf and soccer.

Helen Keller contracted an illness when she was nineteen months old that left her deaf and blind. Yet she became one of the most celebrated, prolific authors, political activists, educators, and humanitarians of the twentieth century.

These examples demonstrate that a soul can rise beyond its limitations and difficulties to live fully, and inspire, touch, and transform others.

Experiencing Déjà Vu

Occasionally, the places you go to or the people you meet can feel so familiar that you may have a strong sense of déjà vu. This often occurs because your soul wants you to pay attention to what is happening around you. Prior to taking on human form, a soul can elect to experience snippets of future events in a particular human body before deciding if it's is the right body to achieve its purpose. Souls can also choose to practice connecting to people and places, or make important decisions while still in the spirit world, in order to give themselves the best chance to carry them out in the physical.

Be Open to Finding Your Purpose

You discover your purpose when you are willing to stop saying that you don't know your purpose and then allow yourself to find out. Examine the thoughts, beliefs, and emotional patterns that do not serve you in your life, and let them go. Think of this as cleaning your house. For instance, does it really serve you to blame others or make them wrong? Can thinking in a limiting way make you happy and successful?

The question of your soul purpose is not so much about a job you do (although that could be part of your life purpose) but about how you live your life. Are you willing to be courageous, sensitive, loving, gentle, and compassionate, and take risks; or will you choose to live your life from a limited perspective of safety and dissatisfaction, where there is little or no room to grow? Will you examine your vulnerabilities, learn to forgive, heal your pain, face your fears, and move forward; or will you spend your life blaming everything and everyone, and resign yourself to a life of limitation, pain, and struggle? In other words, will you look beyond the obvious and explore what is mysterious, unexplained, and extraordinary; or will you narrow-mindedly stick with what you know?

You have the ability to change your mind to see things from a different perspective, allowing things to come into your life rather than struggling. Wisdom can come to you through listening to the radio, watching television, surfing the internet, walking down the street, bumping into a person who inspires you, being given a book, doing something creative, hearing a song that gives you a brilliant idea, meditating, or even having one of your guides or an angel appear in front of you. The main thing is that you need to be open and receptive to signs, your intuition, and déjà vu.

Even an event that you may not consider positive (such as a bad accident or an illness), can lead you to discover your path and contribution in life. Consider the story of an American man who lost his leg during the war, then many years later, read about twin boys from Russia who both had one leg amputated. Because of his own experience, he decided to adopt them and give them a chance of a better life.

Simple Acts

I have discovered that sometimes the simplest acts—a smile, a kind word, or a friendly gesture—can be considered an important contribution that has been made to others. It seems that some of the things that we value highly, such as accumulating a lot of money or being famous, are not necessarily related to what is important to the soul. However, being of service is always significant.

Calling on Higher Guidance

Each person has spirit guides, who are assigned to provide support and assistance. These guides work silently, doing what they can to help you live your life purpose and rarely interfering—unless you ask for help or have an agreement that was made to wake you up, or to encourage you to grow and move forward at a specific time.

Many people become disenchanted with Divine helpers because they are disturbed by all the terrible ways that certain humans behave. What they forget is that we have free will, which gives us an opportunity to learn and grow from our challenges and mistakes. But it is always up to each individual to make their best choices. This is why, instead of blaming Divinity for our lot in life, we should praise our chance to work with higher help hand in hand, to make our lives as empowering and as satisfying as possible.

From my explorations, I have come to understand that spiritual guides want you to ask them for help in all areas of your life. In fact, I encourage people to develop a daily practice of inviting Divine intervention into every area of their life.

You know a spirit guide is helping you when synchronicities occur in your life, you receive information in your mind that is different from your usual thinking, or all of a sudden, you know the solution to a problem. Spirit guides can help you through prophetic dreams, visions, and intuitive guidance, where you can hear a guide's voice telling you to do something or warning you against taking certain actions. You may also become calm in a stressful or traumatic situation and perform the tasks you need to do without thinking about them. Guides can direct you to look up a certain reference book, find a website that answers your questions, or encourage you to call someone who can help you.

My Story: My Soul's Purpose

After I began teaching people how to heal themselves, increase their intuition, and transform their lives, I myself had a very peculiar experience that confirmed my soul purpose.

Having successfully taught my first Visionary Intuitive Healing® workshop, I decided to rest and read a book about Edgar Cayce, an amazing seer who could diagnose illnesses he had never studied and outline treatments he had never heard of. Cayce, called the "sleeping prophet," gave psychic and medical readings to thousands of seekers while in an unconscious state for more than forty years. Cayce died in 1945, at age sixty-seven.

I was relaxing and enjoying reading about Edgar's experiences in the early 1900s when I came to the part where an angel appeared to him. My interest intensified as I read that the angel asked Cayce, who was thirteen, what he wanted more than anything in his life. Edgar said he wanted to help people—especially children—heal. The angel promised that his desire would come true.

As I quietly contemplated what I had read, I thought, *I would love it if an angel appeared to me and told me my soul purpose*. Although I felt that I was on track, I still wanted guidance and confirmation. Within moments of having this thought, I felt a powerful presence in the room.

A magnificent angel appeared in front of me, and I felt its soft waves of warm, healing energy surround me. The angel told me that my role was to remind people to open their hearts, souls, and minds to love, compassion, kindness, and truth. The angel said I was to travel the world and inspire others to get in touch with their own healing ability, intuition, Divine Wisdom, and soul purpose. It explained that I had made a soul agreement to impact, touch, and make a difference in millions of lives all over the world, through my courses, books, articles, and television appearances.

As you can imagine, I was overwhelmed. I had just turned twenty-five, and although I had been seeing clients and teaching personal development workshops since my early twenties, I had no idea how I could achieve what the angel predicted.

The angel said that I would have a lot of help and be guided on my journey. When I pressed for more information, I was told not to worry, that I would gain media exposure and my work would become well known. The angel emphasized that I would first start teaching around Australia, and then overseas. Lastly, I felt embraced by a warm, loving energy and heard, "Don't be concerned; you will be guided and everything will happen perfectly. Just trust." I thanked the angel as it disappeared.

Although I was enthusiastic about my angelic experience, doubt and skepticism began to seep into my mind. It sounded like wishful thinking; after all, I had two small children and had not even traveled out of my home state by myself. I began to question my own sanity and thought I'd made the whole thing up. The only person I told was Paul.

To my surprise, Paul, who can be very skeptical, felt confident that what the angel had predicted would occur.

This was a Saturday morning, and by the evening, I had pretty much forgotten about the angel incident. We were having dinner with a friend when, at about 9 PM, the phone rang. I was contemplating whether I should answer it, convinced that it was my mother calling, but for some peculiar reason the call did not go to our answering machine. I picked up the receiver and said hello. The female voice on the other end told me that I was speaking to a journalist from *Woman's Day*, the largest-selling women's magazine in Australia. I couldn't believe my ears. Could it be possible that the angel was right? I discovered that the journalist was based in Sydney, another synchronicity. For the first time in five years, Paul and I were going to Sydney the following week.

After a chat about healing, she and I decided to meet. As I was about to hang up, she said, "By the way, do you work with angels?" I was truly stunned.

The following Saturday, I was interviewed in Sydney. Afterward, the journalist told me she had intuitive abilities and asked if she could give me a message. I agreed, and she proceeded to tell me that, while speaking to me on the phone, she kept getting a message: "TV, TV, TV."

"You are going to be on TV," she said. I immediately thought of the angel.

Things were certainly becoming interesting. Within a few weeks, I appeared on a major television show and guided people through a self-healing process. Over 40,000 people went to my website and downloaded the self-healing exercise I had shared. Within days, numerous people contacted me and told me that they had been praying for some help when they were guided to turn on the television while I was on. Many had experienced amazing healings during the program and then used the self-healing process to help their family, or to deepen their own healing.

My television appearance and the article in *Woman's Day* opened the doors for me to travel out of state and eventually overseas. Soon after, I was a guest on a number of other shows, and I eventually became a segment presenter and host. This created amazing opportunities for sharing my message of self-healing, love, and the importance of developing your intuition. I am incredibly grateful to the angel for appearing to me that day, strengthening my faith and guiding me on my journey.

Finding Your Legacy

The great thing about discovering your soul's passion is that you can go on to explore it and create your legacy.

When I interviewed Paulo Coelho, bestselling author of *The Alchemist*, he shared, "Every human being on earth has their duty here, his or her experience, the sharing of their legacy. We need to participate in the sharing of this legacy. Writing is the way I found—my way—of sharing my understanding of the present moment. I do that with love. I do that with some pain also, because the process of opening your soul is a little bit delicate. But I do that, and when I look at the result and see that somehow I can be understood, that gives me the sensation that I am not alone and that I am able to share my soul. And I think that when man does not feel alone and feels part of humankind, he feels somehow fulfilled."[16]

I believe that we all know exactly what we love to do. Think about it for a moment: Why are you interested in the things that fascinate you? Why is it that what inspires you and makes your heart quiver is not the same as what makes your friend's heart sing? The problem is that so many of us have been told that we can't listen to our soul's voice, so we bury our heart's desires and forget that we are capable of being creative, passionate, and ingenious. We then begin to hide behind the belief that we actually don't know what to do. Whenever I hear this, I always ask people, "What if you knew exactly what to do?"

Simply Start

Sometimes, even after a lot of exploration and self-discovery, when you have finally realized what you really want to do, the hardest part is to simply start. Paulo Coelho wanted to write since his childhood; however, he kept meeting obstacles and putting off his dream of writing a book—until he went on a pilgrimage to Santiago.

He says, "When I finished the journey, I sat down and said, 'Either I will keep postponing for the rest of my life, waiting for the right time to do it, or I will quit everything, take all the risks, and start writing.' Even though it was late in my life, I decided it was time to do this—not because, at that moment, I thought I could even publish a book. But I understood that I would be defeated in the purpose of the meaning of my life if I could not at least search for my dreams. If I would finish a book was not as important as if I would at least start it."[17]

The truth is that when you go in search of your dream, you will never know whether you will be seen as a success or a failure, based on other people's standards. What you will know is that you had the faith and the courage to give things a go.

Processes for Discovering Your Soul Purpose

Below are several processes that can help you to discover your soul purpose. It may be helpful to do them regularly over a year to receive more clarity about your soul purpose.

Consider Life's Questions

To discover your soul purpose, pay attention to what is happening in your life. Take a pen and paper (or go to your computer, smartphone, or tablet) and give yourself time to answer the following questions. Be as honest with yourself as possible; the more you are willing to discover the bigger picture, the more opportunities you have to grow. You may even be surprised to discover things about yourself that you did not know.

What have been the strongest experiences in your life?

How did they affect you?

What did you learn from them?

How have you grown, transformed, or expanded from those experiences?

What is meaningful to you?

What service would you love to provide to others?

What do you love doing?

What do you keep doing even when it's challenging?

What inspires you?

What comes naturally to you?

Where does your life flow?

Where do you achieve success without great effort?

If you could describe your life with a song, what would it be?

If you could do a painting of your life, what would it look like?

What are the gaps in your life?

Imagine your life in five years' time: if it develops in the same vein as it is in now, what would you regret and what would you be happy about? What things would you need to change? Asking empowering questions helps you focus and move toward your life purpose with ease and grace. When you ask a question, make sure that it expands rather than limits you, because we always receive answers to our questions.

Notice Synchronicity

Notice when unplanned yet related events occur at the same time. This can be a clue to your purpose in life—especially when things start to fall into place without much effort, and you start to feel joy, inspiration, and connection to your heart. Synchronicity is a way for the universe to show you that you are on the right track. It is a sign to infuse you with confidence and encourage you to keep going.

A simple statement you can repeat is: "Divine Source, help me to gently and easily let go of all situations, beliefs, and challenges that block me from living my soul purpose and opening the doors to my Divine design. With the help of the Divine Source, I now bring into my reality the true desires of my heart, which flow to me under grace in perfect ways. Thank you."

Repeat the word "CLEAR" several times, until you feel lighter.

Meditate for Divine Wisdom

Place your hands together in the prayer position and focus on five things you feel grateful for in your life.

While still keeping your thumbs, the heels of your hands, and the tips of your fingers together, slightly bend your fingers. Your hands should resemble the shape of a diamond. If possible, sit down in a meditative position and cross your legs. This position allows you to experience prayer with your soul rather than with words.

Hold your hands in this position in front of your forehead. Look through the opening without blinking your eyes for as long as you can. Then place your hands just above the level of your heart, while holding the same gesture.

Focus on your breathing. Each time you breathe out, focus on the sound *Hoooo*. Hold the sound for as long as you feel comfortable, and allow yourself to move into the invisible world of infinite love, joy and possibilities. Do this for a few minutes.

Place your hands on your heart and allow your own sacred sound to come out. Let your soul sing through you.

When you have completed this process, stand up and focus on your feet. Visualize as golden, reddish rays move through your body and ground you to the earth. Feel your feet on the ground as you reconnect with your mind, body, and soul. Focus your intention on being connected with your whole self.

PART III

TRANSFORMING YOUR LIFE'S RELATIONSHIPS

As you learn to tune in and become conscious of your internal world, reclaim your inner power, and develop your soul's stamina, you have an opportunity to apply what you have learned to your physical reality.

This part of the book explores how you can transform, invigorate, and heal your relationship with yourself, other people, money, and your environment.

While you may decide that the theme of a particular chapter may not be relevant to you, I still urge you to read that section, as you may learn important information that can help you understand yourself, your partner, your parents, your children, or your friends better. Some of the processes could also be pertinent to your present situation, even though the topic may not necessarily interest you.

13

HOW YOU CAN ATTRACT A LOVING PARTNER INTO YOUR LIFE

How do I attract a loving partner into my life? I have heard that you have to
be clear and ask for exactly what you want, so I have made a list of everything I
would like in a partner. However, the people I meet don't seem to match my list,
and I'm beginning to feel extremely frustrated. I'm really tired of being alone,
and I believe I am ready to meet the right person.

In this chapter, I invite you to look within and become conscious of your positive
qualities, which can help you to attract a wonderful mate. I also encourage you to
expand your ideas about love and share processes that can help you to open your heart
to others.

To Attract Love, Be the Loving Partner

In order to attract a loving partner into your life, you must first be the loving partner
you are searching for. Many people desire to find someone who will save them from
themselves and make them happy. They judge and criticize themselves harshly, and
then expect to meet a person who will see past all their unresolved issues, insecurities,
and limitations and love them unconditionally.

Unfortunately, feeling bad about yourself is not very attractive and often draws to
you the exact opposite of what you desire. Each person emanates an energetic field,
which attracts what this person believes he or she deserves. If, deep down, a person

feels unlovable, they are likely to fail to find someone, or attract a person who will prove this belief.

In fact, until you become more loving and complete within yourself, you are likely to keep missing the perfect person for you, even if this person is standing right in front of you. This is because your vibration of feeling bad about yourself does not match his or her vibration of feeling good about themselves. Unless you would like to attract someone who feels incomplete, and is full of insecurities and heavy baggage, you need to work on yourself.

Since, in reality, no one can save you or make you happy long term, your major relationship ought to be with yourself. You need to come into alignment with your deeper essence and begin appreciating who you really are before you can attract a meaningful and satisfying relationship with another person. If you feel whole and complete within yourself—without the need for someone to save you from loneliness, discontent, or suffering—the quality of people you will attract and the experiences you will have are likely to be expansive, inspiring, and uplifting. This way, you are not making someone else responsible for your well-being, so your relationship can be one of freedom, fun, and lightness rather than dependency, control, and neediness. You are also more likely to recognize when a relationship is healthy and empowering rather than one sided, draining, and restricting.

If you are carrying pain from your childhood, then it is really important that you work on your inner child and forgive your parents. Holding on to outdated beliefs and behaviors that your parents demonstrated only keeps you stuck in the past and alone, or attracting the wrong people.

The happier you feel within yourself, the faster you will attract a great person. And I say great, rather than perfect, because no matter what partner you have, he or she will challenge and inspire you at different moments.

Clara's Story: Healing Unconscious Patterns

Clara, a nurse in her mid-thirties, came to see me because she wanted to find Mr. Right. Clara was always moving in and out of unfulfilling relation-

170

ships. During our first meeting, she brought a list of all the qualities she wanted in a man: faithful, reliable, devoted, and honest. This was interesting because, in her relationships with men, Clara lied, often dated more than one man at a time, was unreliable, and was frequently hurtful. I told her that until she was willing to treat others the way she wanted to be treated, she would not find a satisfying relationship.

Clara came from a broken home where her father abused her mother and sister, so her deep-seated belief was that all men were bastards and deserved to be punished. I worked with Clara to heal her childhood trauma and change her beliefs about men. Although it took some time, Clara reemerged feeling better about herself and with a willingness to give men a chance. Even though she felt more vulnerable, Clara opened her heart and met a sensitive man who was able to show her that men can be loving, kind, loyal, generous, and soft. In fact, he was able to completely match Clara's new vulnerability and openness.

Show Love for Yourself

Instead of focusing on what you don't have, start paying attention to all the things you love about yourself. While you are single, take the time to get to know yourself. Ask: *What is unique, amazing, and special about me? What makes me an appealing person? How flexible am I in my life? Am I living my life to the fullest, moving toward my dreams, and being creative; or am I stuck, waiting to be swept off my feet by the ideal person?*

Treat Yourself

I once read a story of a woman who decided that she was going to treat herself with the same love and appreciation she wanted from a man. She would wake up, look in the mirror, and compliment herself on how she looked. Whenever she did something positive in her business, she would congratulate herself. On the weekends, she would take herself out to the theatres, movies, ballet, concerts, and any other events she was interested in. Every day after work, she would have a relaxing bath, dress nicely, and make herself a delicious dinner. She would also set the table with flowers and her best china, and eat by candlelight.

In the beginning, she admitted to feeling a bit silly making all this fuss, but then she realized that she enjoyed it, and it was a lot of fun. Within weeks, she met a wonderful man that she is now in a loving relationship with, who treats her with a lot of care and respect.

Develop Your Abilities

Even if you don't feel that you have the qualities you desire in a partner, look for how you may possess these traits in small quantities. For instance, if finding someone with a sense of humor is important to you but you don't feel that you have a great sense of humor, you may decide to develop it by going to comedy shows, reading joke books, and watching funny movies. In order to be more flexible, you may also go to stand-up comedy shows that you would not usually go to.

Sarah's Story: Releasing Past Hurt

Sarah had not been in a relationship with a man for eight years. She was tall, beautiful, independent, and generous, so it was strange to me that she could not find a partner. I asked Sarah if there were any men she found attractive, and she said yes, but that they appeared frightened of her and unresponsive.

Sarah had felt deeply hurt by her son's father and carried this wound. I encouraged Sarah to attend a healing workshop to release some of her old hurts and discover what could block her from a loving relationship.

During a meditation where we were focusing on the heart center, Sarah saw an image of a vicious spider. When she intuitively inquired what this image meant, she discovered that this invisible spider was protecting her heart and not allowing any man to get close. Although Sarah found this image amusing, she understood the reason why men seemed frightened. In her imagination, Sarah thanked the spider and released it. She then focused on letting go of any hurt, heaviness, and darkness from her heart, and surrounded her heart with pink and green lights, which are powerful for healing the heart. She also gave her heart permission to find the perfect man.

Sarah realized that her heart was the best judge in finding her the right partner. Since her heart had been hurt, it would know how to direct Sarah to a new and empowering experience. She just needed to start trusting its wisdom.

The next day, Sarah felt a strong desire to be in nature. It was a nice day, and she decided to go to one of her favorite city parks. She then walked in a leisurely manner, enjoying the scent of the trees and flowers. After a while, she felt drawn to sit on a bench, next to an attractive gentleman. As it turned out, James had been watching Sarah from a distance. They started to talk and realized they had a lot in common.

Within a month, Sarah and James were nearly inseparable, spending a lot of time together, sharing romantic weekends, and going on overseas trips. James was constantly trying to surprise Sarah and outdo himself. One day, he went to a pharmacy and bought everything he needed to give Sarah a pedicure—never mind that he had never done a pedicure! It was extremely romantic. I was happy to hear that Sarah had opened her heart to a loving relationship, full of creativity and spontaneity.

Open Yourself to Love

Often, we attract people into our lives when we feel happy with ourselves and open to a new adventure. It is important to see people freshly, without judging them or comparing them to our past relationships.

If you've had one or more turbulent relationships in the past, you need to examine if your beliefs and experiences about your former partners are stopping your from meeting someone new. Although it is important to be clear about what you want, you also need to be flexible, as there are no perfect people; just people who are perfect for you. Every relationship has its blessings and challenges. So, make sure that you are not relying on a partner to make you happy; focus on becoming as happy as possible within yourself.

If you feel lonely, go out, find an interesting hobby, and learn to have more fun.

Be Open to Meeting People

Often, I hear complaints from people about the difficulty of finding someone. But this is an opportunity to be intuitive, creative, and open to new experiences. I have heard stories of people feeling an intense desire to go to a particular country, and meeting a soul mate in the strangest place possible.

Several of my friends have found their partners through online dating websites or through other dating services. If you are feeling a bit lost, there is nothing wrong with asking for help. In fact, you might even want to learn some skills for dating and attracting the one you want. Paul has actually cowritten a book with Katia Loisel-Furey, who is a good friend and an expert on the subject of flirting, dating, sex, and love: *How to Get the Man You Want, How to Get the Woman You Want*. This book has fantastic ideas on how to attract that special someone.

Edward's Story: A Little Help

Edward, in his early thirties, was ready to find a woman he could have a long-term relationship with. However, Edward was fairly shy and had limited experience with relationships. In fact, his family was beginning to worry.

Edward was not particularly enthusiastic about coming to a course to learn some skills about attracting a partner; however, with some strategic persuasion, he agreed. Although he seemed content to participate in all the exercises on the first day of the workshop, he was quite reluctant to return for the second day. He made an excuse that he had to play soccer. While it is important to keep prior commitments, the truth was that Edward could play soccer any week. This was an opportunity to change his life.

We knew that there could be some resistance, as people often try to find ways to sabotage new opportunities when they feel uncomfortable. After a little more persuasion, however, Edward agreed to come to the second day of the workshop.

What Edward failed to mention was that he was attracted to Megan, a young woman in the seminar, who he felt was absolutely gorgeous. However, that first day Edward made up his mind that Megan could never like him. So in his reality, there was no point returning. On the second day of the workshop, I discovered Edward's feelings for Megan and encouraged him to make a move. He did.

As it turned out, Megan liked Edward too! And now they are happily married, with a daughter.

Some Interesting Facts

During the process of helping Paul and Katia research their book on getting the one you want, we conducted a study of 504 single men and 498 single women from a variety of backgrounds and social standings, ranging from age twenty-two to fifty-three. Their answers were fascinating! I would like to share a few of the findings with you.

71 percent of men said that romance was more important than sex

96 percent of women said that love is more important than money

100 percent of men said that it was more important that a woman shows him affection than buys him gifts

70 percent of women said they thought a man wasn't interested only to find out that he was flirting

65 percent of men said that they'd avoided eye contact or ignored someone they were attracted to

93 percent of women said that if a man was interested, he should approach the woman of interest

95 percent of men said that women should ask men out

Let Go of Limiting Beliefs about Love

I'd like to encourage you to let go of the idea that only one person or partner can take care of all your needs and desires, and make you feel happy, loved, and fulfilled.

I want to explore this myth because you might be someone who may never find that one person who satisfies you on all levels. Some who are reading this will not have a long-term romantic relationship in this life, and some are already in a relationship in which they can only share certain aspects of their lives and themselves—not necessarily because the person they are with is not for them, but because they may have different interests and values. While spiritual evolution may be an interesting and valuable subject to you, your present or potential partner may be more interested in raising children or playing sports. However, your partner might be completely compatible with you in terms of your appreciation of art, how you deal with your finances, or your travel dreams.

Humanity has tried to sell a very limiting and restrictive idea of love. Basically, we are encouraged to romantically love our partners and share our hearts with them, love our family and our kids, and like our friends, often in a fairly superficial way, with a few exceptions.

Human beings are deeply fearful of closeness and of opening their hearts to a person they cannot define or put into a category of a romantic relationship. Thus, we have a lot of marriages and relationships that either don't work or make people feel like prisoners.

I believe we are entering a time where the strict boundaries of love are becoming blurry. We are beginning to recognize that we need different people and experiences to open our hearts and enrich our lives. We are coming to a point in human evolution where we no longer have to place unrealistic expectations on the person we are with, and expect him or her to meet all our needs.

As we mature as a society, we will stop judging love and allow ourselves and those we care about to develop deep, satisfying connections with a variety of people. Thus, we will allow our hearts to grow, and enter into an experience of love with wisdom, freedom, and respect rather than rules, conditions, and control. We will give ourselves and others the chance to explore and experience deep connections without the need to judge

176

harshly, express jealousy, or make them feel guilty because they may desire more than we can offer. Instead, we will realize that there are many incredible people on earth who have a lot of love, wisdom, and inspiration to offer us. By opening our hearts, we greatly evolve and grow. It is also important to note that these experiences will most likely enhance our primary relationship, creating happiness and contentment in our lives as we feel free to play, explore, and grow.

We need to realize that our partner is not ours; we do not own that person. We have simply come together to share, learn, evolve, and support each other through the good and the challenging times. We also need to understand each other's values, dreams, and desires, and find ways to give each other the freedom to grow.

I believe that the greatest gift we can offer ourselves and others is to live a full, joyful, interesting, inspired life. I have learned that there is no black and white in any relationship, only colors.

Processes for Attracting a Loving Partner

Below are several processes that can help you to attract a loving partner. I suggest that you practice them regularly for the best results; do the process for visualizing and attracting a partner.

Write Down the Qualities You Would Love

Write down the qualities you would love in a partner. Write next to each quality whether you feel you possess the trait you are searching for. If you would like to be with someone who is loving, ask yourself if you are loving; if you want someone who is ambitious and successful, check if you feel ambitious and successful; if you desire someone generous, fun, vibrant, and healthy, then make sure that you are a match.

Work on Your Heart

Working on your heart and releasing any stuck energies is vital. Place your hands on your heart, and take some slow, deep breaths. Become aware of whether your heart feels open, relaxed, and soft, or tense, protected and afraid.

If your heart is tense and afraid, acknowledge those feelings. Ask yourself if you are holding on to past experiences that have caused you pain. Allow memories of these experiences to come to the surface. Reflect on these experiences. What decision did you make based on the hurt you felt? How long ago did these experiences occur? Is the pain serving you now? What positive things came out of these challenges? What did you learn? How did you grow?

By keeping your heart closed, what potential experiences are you missing out on? What excuses do you use to keep yourself limited and alone?

If the experiences that are repeating again and again in your life are not working for you, you need to recognize the patterns that are recurring, and the limiting beliefs and feelings you are holding on to, and change them.

Find an Example

Find an example of people who have fantastic relationships and interview them. Discover what works for them and why.

Visualize Attracting a Partner

Rub your hands together, making sure you rub each finger. Imagine that you have a beautiful pink ball of light between your hands, and focus on intensifying its energy. Think of as many loving, positive things about yourself as you can for thirty seconds.

Place your hands in front of your heart, move them in a circular motion, and take a couple of deep breaths. Imagine that your heart is opening and growing. Do this for thirty to forty seconds.

Relax your hands.

Be willing to risk opening your heart and trust that you can attract into your life a person who complements, supports, and deeply enriches your life.

Say an Invoking Statement.

Say: "Divine Love, assist me to heal any past hurts that have scared me and are keeping me stuck. Please help me to release any negative, limiting, or burdensome beliefs, feelings, and memories that I am carrying, which are preventing me from recognizing my own worth and attracting a loving, caring partner into my life. Allow me to experience deep love in my heart and to share this love with a partner who will appreciate, enjoy, and grow with me."

Repeat the word "CLEAR" several times, until you feel lighter.

Focus Your Intention

Close your eyes. Think of all the great qualities you have. Imagine listing those qualities on a golden sheet of paper. Now visualize a golden-red bubble of light in front of you, and place the list in it.

On another sheet of golden paper, imagine writing down a list of all the qualities you would love in a partner. Include everything you would like this person to have. Make sure you mention that your perfect partner needs to be single and available. (Sometimes a person can be single but married to their job, which makes a relationship difficult or almost impossible.) Place this list into the golden-red bubble.

Imagine gently allowing the bubble to float away into the universe, toward your perfect mate. Allow yourself to feel your heart open and connect to his or her heart. Sense how the love from your heart re-energizes this person's heart and how the love from their heart re-energizes yours. Allow yourself to rejoice about having created this connection, which will draw you two to each other in the most perfect way, at the most ideal time, with ease and grace.

Trust that your request has been heard. Find ways to enjoy yourself, and feel good about your life.

14

HOW YOU CAN CREATE HARMONY
IN YOUR RELATIONSHIP

My partner of many years is very negative and drains my energy.
We have different beliefs, interests, and ideas about life. I have changed many
things in my life and am beginning to really enjoy myself, and feel creative.
However, my husband's attitude really upsets me, and I don't know if there
is a way to improve our relationship and make it harmonious,
or if the healthiest solution is to separate.

Before we can create harmony in a relationship, we need to experience peace within ourselves. It is extremely easy to blame other people for our lack of inner contentment. Every person we are close to in our life gives us an opportunity to know ourselves better and to practice inner stillness in the face of challenge. This practice builds our emotional and spiritual stamina, and expands our nervous system so that we can handle a higher influx of information without being overwhelmed.

Taking a Different Point of View

Conflicts in relationships usually arise when both parties are so caught up in their own points of view and ideas about life that they stop taking the time to listen to, connect to, and grow with each other. Someone who has lived with his or her partner for an extended period of time often creates assumptions about that person, instead of discovering who they are on a daily basis. The best way you can help your partner change is to take an expanded perspective and give your partner the space to adjust. For instance, if you place a person in an environment where others treat them as a success, that person is much more likely to triumph than if you put the same person in a situation where failure is expected.

Having Compassion

Compassion, softness, and a balanced point of view can do wonders for rejuvenating a stale relationship.

If it bothers you that your partner is negative and you're committed to healing your life, you may need to check within yourself where you are negative and refuse to admit it. We have all heard the saying, "Whatever we resist persists." Do you always try to be positive in your life, or are you aware that you express yourself in an aggressive way at times? Are you always nice, or do you get frustrated and complain to others about your struggles? The more you recognize these unlikable qualities in yourself, the faster you can forgive others while allowing them to have the freedom to express all aspects of themselves, without you being upset or drained.

At times, it can be difficult to understand another person until you walk in his or her shoes. One of the most important things I learned when I was studying acting was how to experience the world from the point of view of the character I was playing. This has helped tremendously to understand the thoughts, emotions, behavioral patterns, and actions of others.

If you let go of needing to be right and become more compassionate toward others, then they will stop reacting negatively to you and start listening. The more charged and stressed you are about an issue, the more likely people will resist you.

A balanced point of view can give you the clarity to communicate with your partner without trying to control, judge, or agitate. You need to discover your partner's highest values and embrace them. If your mate's highest value is family, and he or she feels that the changes you are making might compromise your love, care, affection, and support, then fear and defiance are normal. However, if you assure your partner that your transformation will bring more love, time, and enjoyment, they may change their tune and become interested in supporting you on your journey.

Focus on the Positive Aspects

If you are in a relationship that you feel you can improve, start focusing on all the positive aspects of your partner.

First, acknowledge all that you love about him or her. Really feel your appreciation for what your partner does—how they make you feel good, happy, cared for, attractive, and so forth. If you are not currently feeling amenable toward your partner, then remember times in the past when you did and draw upon these memories to help you be more receptive. Then encourage your partner by sharing your positive feelings. This can be as simple as saying, "I really liked how you kissed me today; I am grateful that you went shopping and bought some food; thank you for taking the time to call me; I love the way you look in that shirt; the dinner you made was delicious," and so on.

Emphasize the positives rather than saying, "I'm so annoyed that you didn't do the dishes, take out the trash, and feed the cat." Everybody likes positive reinforcement. It motivates people and creates pleasant, relaxing sensations inside the body. Wouldn't you rather have someone encourage you than criticize you?

Learn the Various Expressions of Love that Work

There are a variety of expressions of love; discover them. What is loving to one person may not be to another. If you know what each of you love, you can create a much stronger bond.

For instance, women often need time to talk and share how they are feeling. When they share, they rarely want a man to fix a problem; their desire is to be heard. Men can get agitated when they feel that their advice is not welcome.

One way around this challenge is to tell a man: "I feel like I would love to share something with you, and it may take ten to fifteen minutes. I don't really want you to help me; I just want you to listen and empathize." This can help him relax and listen.

Men often need space and quiet time to regenerate, so it is important to give a man room to breathe. Sporting activities offer another great way for many men to release pressure, tension, and frustration.

The idea is to encourage, understand, and complement each other. Questions you might explore include: "What is my mate's highest potential? How can I support him or her in manifesting it?" Of course, it is important to find out from your partner what their present interests and goals are.

You may also decide to explore what you and your partner need to feel loved. For instance, are you someone who needs sweet, loving, affirmative words to feel cared about? Or do you love physical touch and affection? Maybe surprises, romantic dinners, poems, love notes, mysterious trips, special gifts, and unexpected serenades thrill you? Your partner, on the other hand, might feel special when you take time to be fully present, relaxed, and do something they love with the phone turned off and no interruptions. Perhaps helping your mate with the household chores, shopping, or looking after the kids will make him or her feel appreciated and treasured. Learning what makes your partner tick can be the difference between an extraordinarily delicious relationship and a tired, mediocre one.

We are all more capable of passionate, intimate, sensual, unconditional love than we give ourselves credit for. The truth is, to master any relationship to a high degree of love and connection requires effort, practice, consideration, appreciation, empathy, wisdom, kindness, softness, and growth, as well as the willingness to listen and communicate.

In other words, instead of trying to prove who is right, more valuable, or works harder, find what is lovable about each person, focus on gratitude, and ask each other how you can make your life together more joyful. Letting go of control, listening, and becoming flexible in a relationship can make all the difference.

When a Relationship Is Destructive

In order for a relationship to work, both partners must invest time, love, connection, honesty, creativity, and energy. Although one-way partnerships can be tolerable for short periods, they often bring numbness, frustration, isolation, and suffering. Communication is the key to any healthy relationship.

It is possible for a couple to have diverse interests and still live in harmony with each other if they are willing to honor and respect each other's differences. However, they need to find a language that allows them to understand and nurture one another.

If your partner is abusive and only wants things his or her own way, and no amount of communication, appreciation, or compassion changes the harmful behavior, then you need to consider what your life is worth and whether leaving could be the best solution. And if you do separate, it is vitally important that you work on yourself to understand what lessons you needed to learn in your last relationship, so that you do not attract the same experience again.

Helen's Story: From Victim to Empowered, Courageous Woman

Helen emailed me with a desperate plea for help to save her marriage. So we organized a distance healing session, as she lives in Europe. Helen called me on Skype and shared that her husband was considering a divorce. She felt distraught at the idea.

Helen and Trevor had been married for over twenty years and had an eighteen-year-old son. Trevor was an important public figure, often traveling. When they were married for just over a year, Helen found a love letter in Trevor's jacket. She confronted him, but he just brushed her off.

Helen felt rejected and betrayed. Her body reacted violently, and she developed rashes all over. Trevor did not notice. From that moment, Helen had to force herself to have sex with Trevor, who often told her she was ugly and useless. As Helen had no family to turn to, she just accepted the abuse. When she became pregnant, Trevor wanted Helen to abort the child, but Helen insisted on having the baby. She felt like that was her opportunity to love and be loved.

Trevor became a little softer after the baby was born. He decided that he liked the idea of having a son, although it was Helen's job to look after him. One day, while playing with her son in the park, Helen met Jerome. Like her husband, Jerome was a difficult, complex man, but he paid attention to her, showing her some warmth and love. Jerome and Helen had an affair for six years. However, because her husband provided financial support, the idea of leaving him was incomprehensible. Helen also had a deep terror of being alone. Although Helen never talked about her affair, she lived in fear of Trevor finding out. Helen developed serious ovarian problems and anxiety. Her body was screaming out. She became ill with chronic fatigue, had a nervous breakdown, and could hardly digest food.

I asked Helen if she and Trevor ever had deep discussions. Helen said that they never really talked, and when they did, it was unpleasant and painful.

As I worked with Helen, I focused on helping her release her guilt, fear, anger, humiliation, and shame. I also assisted her to reconnect with her inner strength and courage. Whenever I tuned in, I had a strong feeling that she could make a huge contribution to society through her creativity. I encouraged Helen to start expressing herself through art and to spend time in nature.

I knew that Helen would not make any hasty decisions and had to become comfortable with the idea that she was valuable and capable of looking after herself. Slowly, Helen began changing how she saw herself. She spent time in nature, wrote, and painted. Her work was eventually published, and she was invited to speak at small gatherings. As Helen began to feel more confident, she changed her hairstyle, bought clothes that flattered her, and started attending various interesting functions. Although she still felt lonely on occasion, most of the time, she felt strong. She was proud of herself for taking important steps forward—from a victim to an empowered, courageous woman.

I shared with Helen that we are often treated by others the way we treat ourselves. This idea had a substantial impact on her, and she became more loving, gentle, and caring with herself, the way she wished Trevor would be.

In the beginning, Trevor felt uncomfortable with Helen's changes, but as time went by, he started to perceive her differently. A new level of respect awakened inside him, and he began paying her a different type of attention.

In fact, Helen told me he started bringing home little gifts, organizing romantic dinners, and for the first time in their marriage, actually listening to her. Trevor even agreed to attend some programs on personal development. During the seminars, Trevor realized how closed he had kept his heart and how badly he had treated Helen.

Trevor and Helen decided that they were willing to forgive and get to know each other again. They were also prepared to work with their shadow parts as they focused on improving their marriage. The idea was that they would be equal partners in the relationship, giving each other the freedom to explore what they needed to while sharing their life together.

Helen tells me that, although it is not always easy, she feels grateful to be with Trevor and proud of their progress.

While Helen and Trevor were able to turn their relationship around and forgive the abuse, there are times when a relationship may have run its course, and the safest and healthiest thing is to leave, particularly if there is any physical violence. If you are facing a dangerous situation, then always seek approriate support.

Processes for Creating Harmony in Relationships

Here are three effective processes for improving your relationship. The cord-clearing process in particular is really powerful, so I suggest you use it regularly to clear energy between yourself and your partner, as well as other people you are close to.

Take a New Point of View

If you would like to improve the relationship with your partner, imagine swapping places and looking at the situation from his or her perspective. How do things look? Can you understand and have compassion? If you could speak in a way they understood, what would you say? Try to let go of your assumptions about your partner and take a fresh look. Be willing to communicate, and find out what your partner thinks and feels. Don't assume that you already know. Discover how they want to be loved.

Set an Intention

Say: "Divine Healing Intelligence, please help me to release any anger, righteous attitude, resentment, limited point of view, and _____ [add anything else you feel] that I am holding onto about _____ [put in the name of the person and what upsets you about what they do]. I am willing to start fresh and discover the positive potential in _____ [put in the name of the person].

Help me see, feel, and experience harmony, understanding, care, and love in this relationship. Please help us to resolve our differences and be open to listening, hearing, and supporting each other. I am now willing to experience and appreciate all the positive qualities my partner possesses. Thank you."

Repeat the word "CLEAR" several times, until you feel lighter.

Perform a Cord Clearing

Although a lot of people have been taught to cut or sever cords or ties, I don't believe that it is a healthy practice: first, because you cannot slice energy; and second, because even the intention of cutting the cord can reawaken your birth trauma, when the cord between you and your mother was severed. From experience, I believe that the gentlest and kindest way to transform a challenging relationship is to release any negativity from the cords, and then, through color and intention, infuse healthy, positive energy. This is a simplified version of a very powerful and effective process I teach in my workshops to transform difficult relationships. Use it with your partner when you feel that you are misunderstanding each other, or are feeling frustrated or angry with each other.

Imagine that there is an energetic cord that is attached from your solar plexus energy center to your partner's. If you could tune in to it, what would this cord look like? Would it be thick, heavy, and twisted or light, clear, and thin? If there were energy inside it, would it be positive energy or heavy, negative energy?

If the energy feels unhealthy, imagine a powerful, golden ray of light flowing into your solar plexus and moving into the cord, clearing all the density out of your half of the cord to the middle, where your half of the cord connects with your mate's half. Imagine that the cord opens in the middle, and all the negative energy that you have been holding releases into a violet fire. Then visualize the gold light flowing into your partner's solar plexus and clearing all the density, hurt, anger, or frustration that they are carrying in relation to you. Imagine that this gold light moves all the dense energy into the middle, where all the negativity dissolves into the violet flame, and then the fire is extinguished. Violet is a great color to transmute dense and negative energy.

Focus on sending love, peace, and care into the cord, and observe as it assimilates into the gold light that circulates between you and your partner. The color can also change to green, which shows healing, especially related to issues of the heart; pink, which demonstrates that love and care is flowing through the cord; or purple, which strengthens your spiritual connection.

After you have cleared the cords, focus on all the positive qualities your partner has. Focus on your partner's potential instead of weaknesses. See your partner succeed in whatever area he or she feels challenged. You can ask yourself: *What positive action has my partner done today that I can acknowledge and appreciate?* Write down these actions or reflect on them in your mind. Then share them with your partner. Visualize your partner responding positively to you.

15

HOW YOU CAN PREPARE YOUR BODY FOR PREGNANCY

I would really love to get pregnant and have heard that there are things
I can do to prepare my body for pregnancy. I would also like to know if I can
communicate with the soul of my baby before he or she is born.
I would love to have a natural birth. Do you have any tips?

If you and your partner plan to have children or are in the midst of a pregnancy, this chapter can help you connect with your baby, work on resolving past issues, and explore natural birth. Even if you are not pregnant or have no intention of having children, you may like to read this section to deepen your understanding of your own birth, and whether some of your deepest beliefs are your own or come from your parents. It is important to emphasize that recognizing that you are carrying someone else's pain or beliefs can help you to let go and move forward, rather than blame your parents for your experience.

Taking Time to Prepare

Having children is a very serious decision, and it's important to prepare mentally, emotionally, energetically, and physically for this experience. On a mental level, it's vital that you and your partner have a healthy relationship, and take time to communicate with each other. At times, unresolved issues in a relationship can make it difficult for a woman to get pregnant, as subconsciously, she may not feel it is safe to bring up a child. Occasionally, the pain may stem from a past relationship.

On an emotional level, it is really beneficial to do some internal work on yourself and your childhood, as well as any hurtful relationships from the past, before you become pregnant. You may need to look at forgiving your parents or former partners in order to feel more emotionally stable and comfortable.

If you plan to be a single parent, then you need to make sure you have enough support from your family and friends to take this step. It is also advisable to speak to other single parents to understand exactly what is involved in bringing up a child on your own.

Alexia's Story: Difficulties Conceiving

Alexia came to see me because she was having difficulty conceiving. She had a number of ovarian cysts, and doctors told her she had a very slim chance of getting pregnant. Alexia was distraught, as she was in her mid-thirties and had finally found a man with whom she wanted to spend her life and raise a family.

Deep in her heart, Alexia felt that she could get pregnant. When I was tuning in to her, I could see a little girl in her aura. However, the message I received from her baby's soul was that Alexia needed to release the pain she was carrying from her last relationship. Alexia had been engaged to a man a few years previously; they talked about starting a family and being together until old age. However, days before the wedding, Alexia and her fiancé had a fight, and he called off the wedding.

Alexia was devastated, as it seemed like all her dreams had just vanished. She became reclusive and depressed. Not long after, she discovered that she had ovarian cysts. As I have helped many women who have had cysts, I know that they related to unfulfilled dreams, holding on to regrets, disappointments, failures, and the fear of being hurt. When I read the symptoms to Alexia from my book *The Secret Language of Your Body*, she could relate to most of them.

192

I worked with Alexia to release disappointments from her ex-partner's broken promises and her anxiety around trusting a man again. Alexia also had a deep fear of abandonment, as her mother had died when she was young.

I encouraged Alexia to attend "The Secret Language of Your Body" workshop, where she could learn tools to communicate with and heal her body.

Alexia changed her diet, started to exercise, took helpful supplements, and made time to meditate, connect with and listen to her body, and work on her emotions. She also shared all her concerns with her partner, who was very supportive, and reassured her that he was fully committed to their relationship and was keen to be a father.

I encouraged Alexia to have some acupuncture treatments from a qualified practitioner who helps women prepare for pregnancy and birth. I had a very positive experience with acupuncture when I was pregnant with my daughter, and I cannot recommend it highly enough—as long as you find a highly qualified practitioner.

Within a few months of preparing her body for a baby, Alexia conceived. During her pregnancy, she felt strong, and she gave birth to a healthy girl.

Creating an Optimal State

How a mother feels during her pregnancy has a huge effect on the child and on the way the child lives life. It is essential to make sure that you are in an optimal mental and emotional state during pregnancy and birth. If an emotional or physical challenge arises while you are pregnant, recognize and deal with it in a gentle but swift manner, so that you do not pass any negativity on to the baby. In fact, the ideal situation is to spend as much time as possible focusing on positive, loving, nurturing emotions while you are pregnant, and directing these emotions to your baby.

Listening to beautiful music, while rubbing your belly and sending loving thoughts and images of love, is a powerful way to make a connection with your child, helping him or her feel safe. If you have a partner, encourage them to sing, talk to, and send loving energy to the baby too.

Tim's Story: A Mother's Anxiety

Tim attended my workshop because he didn't know how to deal with his anxiety. During the exercises on communicating with his body, Tim became aware that when he was a fetus in his mother's womb, he had adopted his mother's worries.

During the healing process, Tim realized that his mother's apprehension was her experience, and that, unconsciously, he had been punishing himself for causing her pain and discomfort during the pregnancy. In fact, Tim's mother had a lot of conflict with Tim's father about their finances and survival when she was pregnant. Not surprisingly, Tim always struggled with money.

In the workshop, Tim was able to release the unconscious guilt he carried from the womb and free himself from holding on to his mother's fear. Incredibly, after the process, Tim's anxiety disappeared. When I saw him months later, he looked confident, relaxed, and at peace. He told me that he felt like a different person. He had also been given a promotion at work.

Connecting to the Soul of the Baby

Many women say that they can feel their baby's soul before they even get pregnant. Sometimes they dream about the baby; at other times, they can feel the energy of their child around them. Occasionally, they say they can actually see and communicate with the baby's spirit.

Before I was pregnant with my daughter, Angelina, I got strong images and visions that I would have a daughter soon. When I found out I was pregnant, I felt a bit concerned that it was too soon to have a second child, as I was only twenty-three and already had my son, Raphael, who was two at the time. When I was meditating on what to do, I was shown a beautiful baby girl. She told me that she has chosen me as her mummy, and she was very excited to be my daughter. After that, I felt very comfortable with my decision to have her.

When she was about four years old, Angelina told me that she had been praying and thanking God. When I asked her why, she said, "For giving me a beautiful mummy like you." I was very touched and so grateful to have such a beautiful, loving, and wise child.

Working with Energy Centers

On an energetic level, I often advise my clients to work with their chakras. It is especially beneficial to work on the first, second, and third chakras when preparing the body for pregnancy. Red, orange, and yellow are excellent colors to warm the body and create a receptive environment for the baby. These are also the colors of the first three chakras.

The First Chakra

The first chakra holds all your familial beliefs and patterns. It is linked to support, loyalty, safety, and a sense of oneness. It also contains fears about our physical survival, loss and abandonment, shame, and betrayal. When you connect with this chakra, you may want to examine which beliefs you adopted from your childhood that are no longer legitimate. Do you still have unresolved issues with your family members? Are you willing to heal these relationships? Do you have a fear of abandonment that you are holding on to? Do you keep people at a distance or push them away before they can reject you? As you answer these questions, reflect on whether these beliefs serve you or whether you are ready to let them go.

The Second Chakra

The second chakra relates to your significant relationships. It is linked to external success, choice, honesty, creativity, communion, and sexuality. It also contains fears around survival, lack, failure, control, rejection, and isolation. Here, you may look at what role you play in your relationships. Are you empowered or victimized? Do you feel like a child with money, or are you able to master your finances? How often do you make choices based on money rather than what you would really love to have or do? Can you allow yourself to be creative in your life? How do you feel about your body and sensuality? As you contemplate the answers, ask yourself if you are willing to take more responsibility for your life by taking positive actions.

The Third Chakra

The third chakra is connected to your personal power and self-esteem. It is linked to self-confidence, respect, discipline, courage, and action. It also stores the fear of looking stupid, failing, being seen as unattractive, being criticized, not feeling good enough, and aging. When you connect with this chakra, explore your feelings about yourself. What do you love about yourself? What aspects have you rejected? How important is it for you to please others and have them like you? How much importance do you give to what others think? Do you have the courage to listen to your own wisdom and make the changes you need? How would you know if you were happy?

As a parent, you regularly have to make critical decisions about your children's lives. In order to be a great example to your children, you need to be a courageous and wise explorer of your own life, demonstrating an ability to heal, transform, and lead.

Natasha's Story: Dealing with Loss

Natasha came to my workshop with her husband, Simon, a doctor who practiced integrative medicine. Natasha, eight months pregnant, was terrified of giving birth. Before she had become pregnant, she battled a terrible kidney infection for almost a year, which severely weakened her immune system. Natasha was eager to understand the messages her body was imparting before giving birth.

I told Natasha that, on an emotional level, kidneys hold ancient sadness, regrets, guilt, blame, suffering, the inability to trust, tiredness, and fear. Intuitively, I felt that her kidney problems were connected to her decision to become a mother.

Natasha shared that her mother had died unexpectedly when she was twenty. When this happened, Natasha was so shocked and distressed that, instead of grieving, she pushed away all the pain and buried herself in her studies. Ten years later, when Natasha turned thirty, she felt that she wanted to be a mother.

All the unprocessed pain and grief that Natasha had buried manifested as a kidney infection. Although she no longer had the infection, she still felt a lot of sensitivity and discomfort around her kidneys, and wanted to heal completely. She resonated with my explanation and was willing to do a completion ceremony with her mother.

I advised Natasha to place her hands on the area of her body where she was still holding grief and take slow breaths. I also shared that releasing sorrow would help her baby feel more peaceful and comfortable. Natasha placed her hands on her solar plexus, closed her eyes, and visualized her mum as she remembered her. She talked to her mum, telling her how devastated she felt at her passing. She also imagined that her mum answered. Natasha shared with her mum her feelings about becoming a mother and her disappointment at not having her mum around for the birth. She then asked her mother's soul to bless and support her during labor.

After Natasha completed the process, she felt exhausted but cleansed. All the discomfort she had in her kidneys disappeared. I encouraged her to communicate with her mother whenever she needed extra support, knowing that her mother's love was always there. I also urged Natasha to recognize where female support and motherly influence was present in her life.

During labor, Natasha felt strong, empowered, and supported. She gave birth naturally to a beautiful baby boy.

Natural Birth

Natural birth can be an empowering way to bring a child into the world. And a natural approach is often gentler, less stressful, and less intrusive, with little complication afterward.

A satisfying birth experience is strongly linked to the amount of control a woman feels she can exercise over the actual birth. Preparation is the key to natural birth.

In natural birthing classes, women are taught to use their breath, heat, massage, and water to lessen the pain in labor. They are also encouraged to mentally prepare and use relaxation, visualization, and affirmation techniques to assist themselves through pregnancy, birth, and motherhood. Some women also work with hypnosis, color healing, and aromatherapy to aid them through the process.

To sustain energy during labor, rhythmic beats through music, vocalization, and movement are recommended. Acupuncture is another fantastic tool for increasing energy, speeding up labor, and minimizing the intensity of contractions. Women are encouraged to develop an attitude of surrender, welcoming the labor instead of resisting it. The more the mother is relaxed and informed, the easier she will handle labor, even if it becomes difficult and she requires intervention.

One part of preparation is having a birth plan, which helps a woman understand the different aspects of birth and clarify in her mind what is going to happen. The plan also lists her choices, such as the kind of support she desires during labor and birth, her preferences for pain relief and birth positions, as well as the care she desires after the baby is born.

Water births can provide a very gentle transition for the baby, who moves from water into water, and therefore, does not experience the shock of cold air. Water in labor is tremendously useful in opening and relaxing the mother as well. The experience of weightlessness and warmth helps with pain relief.

Researchers have discovered that postpartum depression is considerably lower in women who have a natural birth. It is important to do the research necessary before you become pregnant and during pregnancy to assure that you have the best possible experience of bringing a new life into this world. Of course, the most important thing is the health of the baby and the mother, so if medical intervention is required, it should always be taken.

Processes for Preparing for Pregnancy

The following are three powerful processes to help you prepare for pregnancy. I suggest you work with the second and third process daily until you become pregnant.

Ask Questions

To prepare yourself for pregnancy, ask: *Am I ready to have this child? Do I have the emotional and financial support required? Is there anything I need to resolve or heal before I am ready to have a baby? Am I physically healthy, or do I need to improve my health? Do I need any extra supplements that can balance my system and make it stronger?*

Meditate to Connect with the Baby

If you feel that you are ready to have a baby, you can do a simple meditation of calling the child's soul toward you: Lie or sit comfortably. Close your eyes, and take slow, deep breaths. Allow your body to relax and unwind. The softer and more relaxed you feel, the better. Imagine a beautiful yellow flame in front of you. Allow the flame to grow bigger and warmer.

Say: "Divine Intelligence, I am ready to be a mother (or father). Please help me connect to the soul of my child."

Take some slow, deep breaths and allow yourself to sense the connection.

Ask to see the child, or simply sense him or her. Surround your child with beautiful pink light. Place your hands on your heart, feel the warmth, and allow the love, gentleness, and support from your heart to connect to this soul. Let this soul know how much you would love to have him or her in your life.

Invite a Child into Your Life

Say: "I invite you into my life. I am willing to love you, take care of you, and support you in your growth and expansion. I ask that, if it is for my highest good and your highest good, you come into my life in perfect time, with ease and grace. Thank you for connecting with me." (Feel free to add anything else.)

Repeat the word "ALLOW" several times, until you feel lighter.

When you are pregnant, feel free to communicate with your child, playing soft music, singing to them, and doing gentle healing exercises.

A Daily Process If You Experience Challenges Getting Pregnant

Rub your hands together for thirty seconds. Visualize a ball of orange light between your hands. In your mind's eye, make it as intense and warm as possible. Breathe deeply and slowly. Place your hands on your lower abdomen where your uterus is situated.

Take a deep breath in and then exhale slowly. Imagine that the orange ball moves through your uterus, and clears any density, stuckness, or negativity out of your uterus, ovaries, and any other related organs. Ask that your uterus create the best possible environment for a baby to grow in. Visualize soft pink light moving through your uterus, and send it vibrations of love and softness. Then imagine a healthy baby growing inside you, feeling happy, joyful, and protected.

Take a few more deep breaths, relax your hands, and gently open your eyes. Focus on honoring your body and being gentle with yourself.

16

How You Can Raise Healthy, Confident Children

I have young children, and I would like to learn ways to assist them
to be more confident and help them heal.

Once you have children, your task is raising them to be healthy, happy, self-assured individuals. Education, time, and love are major keys in helping children feel confident. I encourage you to apply my suggestions though the use of color healing, imagination, and visualization to help your children deal with challenges such as rejection, fears, difficulty sleeping, and a variety of health issues.

Encouraging Healthy Habits in Children

It is important to inspire children to eat in a healthy manner from an early age. Obesity in children is a real problem that can lead to health problems, lack of confidence, and bullying. So take the time to educate them about eating nutritious food. You might decide to take them shopping, cook with them, and teach them what a well-balanced diet is. Another way to make eating fun and healthy is to try to include a variety of colorful food in their diets. If your children are younger, you can create a game of how many colors they can eat at each meal. You can also briefly explain the qualities of each color as they are eating or drinking, so that they feel confident that they are improving their heath and gaining strength as they eat. This can also promote variety and encourage them to try new food.

Touch and Connection

Children require time and attention from their parents. They need to feel loved and be shown a lot of affection to feel happy and healthy. Numerous studies demonstrate that babies who are not touched have weakened immune systems, may suffer severe emotional problems, exhibit violent behavior, have slower development, and are subject to more illnesses.

As adults, we need to take the time to encourage and inspire children to become creative, warm, kind, caring, and responsible. We also need to give children the time and space to dream, play, and discover without pushing them to become what we think they should be.

Understanding Why Children Get Sick

There are no simple or easy answers to the question of why children get sick. In fact, I have always told people that, although we have many similarities, each person is unique and must personally discover the particular factors that create specific conditions in their bodies. I have spent years teaching people to connect with and listen to the wisdom of their bodies. What I've learned is that the state that the mother is in while pregnant, and how she feels about herself, her partner, family, and finances, have a deep influence on the child. This is not to say that we need to blame the mother, or father, for any difficulties the child experienced. However, we do need to develop compassion and an understanding of our bodies, and what causes our bodies to stress and deteriorate.

If we look at the perspective of the soul, we can see the soul choosing a certain body, either because it needs to deal with a particular karmic situation, learn something, or teach others. It is also possible that a parent and a child have previously agreed to a contract, which can only be fulfilled through illness.

Lilly's Story: Illness as Insight into the Past

Through my different travels, I have met many people who have had sick children. My intention has always been to be compassionate with those people, help their children get better, and offer support.

On a trip overseas, I met Lilly, who had a son who had been battling leukemia for several years. From meeting many people who have leukemia, I have gathered that, since it is a blood disorder, it has a lot of relevance to family and blood ties.

When Lilly found out what I did, she asked if I could give her some insights into why her son had developed leukemia. When I tuned in to Lilly, I could feel that she carried a lot of unprocessed pain in relation to her father, who had died two years earlier. I also felt that there had been abuse in the family. Lilly confirmed this, telling me that there had been incest in her family, and a lot of pain and trauma that had never been resolved. Lilly also told me that when she was pregnant with her son, she was experiencing a lot of stress. There were court cases, sicknesses, anger, lies, and resentment. Lilly's father got very ill around that time. So, she was unable to talk to him about all the pain she was carrying. Lilly developed fibromyalgia as well as chronic fatigue as a result of all her stress.

When I shared my insights, Lilly told me that she felt relieved. She understood that her son was trying to process the family issues she was not able to deal with. Instead of blaming herself, Lilly resolved to make changes to her lifestyle and to work on healing her past. As she did, her health improved, and her son slowly recovered with the help of both natural and allopathic support.

Children Are Naturally Receptive to Healing

There are many different approaches and creative ways to help children increase their confidence and discover their natural healing abilities. We need to start teaching children to feel good about themselves as soon as possible. Researchers tell us that the first seven to eight years of a child's life are vitally important in how they will function for the rest of their lives. A child's early experiences play a significant role in their development of physical, social, emotional, and intellectual skills. Developmental neurologists say that the happier a child's experiences are, the more neural connections they create, dramatically enhancing their ability to process and transmit information inside the brain.

Before you are able to teach your child self-healing techniques, you must first gain their trust and make the process fun.

Healing with Color and Creative Visualization

Children are innately open to healing and creative visualization. They are always creating, imagining, and conceiving games, stories, and entertainment for themselves. Color healing is one of the simplest ways to start helping them deal with the challenges of being a child. Color healing can help children feel loved, release tension, give reassurance, create calm, increase self-esteem, improve memory skills, develop creative thinking, fall asleep, and heal various health conditions.

Use the wisdom I have included in this book to make the healing process most effective. In *The Secret Language of Your Body*, there is an entire section on the healing properties of color. It can help you use the colors more effectively. Also, see *The Secret Language of Color Cards* deck, which describes the positive attributes of forty-five colors and also gives short healing processes that you can do.

Although I have mentioned using color to heal physical problems, it is important that you use this information wisely. Color healing works in conjunction with medical and alternative treatments, so please make sure you give your child the best chance to heal by using both when appropriate. Doctors who practice integrative medicine can be fantastic at advising you when it is important to use medicine, as well as when it is valuable to work with other therapies.

Alicia's Story: Color Healing for Fevers

Alice called me because her daughter had a high fever that would not go down. She told me that she did not want to give her medicine, as she'd heard that fevers can help the immune system get rid of infection. She wanted to help her daughter to feel better in a natural way. I told Alice that the best color for reducing a fever is blue, and I encouraged her to ask her daughter to visualize blue bubbles of light moving into her head and body. I also asked Alice to rub her hands together, visualize a big blue ball of energy between them, place an intention of lowering the temperature, and then move her hands above her daughter's body, urging her daughter to take slow, deep breaths.

Alice did as I had instructed and called me an hour later to tell me that her daughter was feeling much better, and her fever had gone.

Raphael and Angelina's Story: Color-Healing Meditation

When my son, Raphael, was about six and my daughter, Angelina, was three and a half, I started teaching them about color healing and meditation. Every night before they went to bed, I asked them to pick a color they liked and told them a little bit about the different qualities that color contained. Then I asked them to close their eyes and imagine themselves being surrounded by the color we discussed. Sometimes we did particular meditations or made up stories involving characters who had magical abilities when using certain colors.

On the nights when I was having difficulty getting Raphael and Angelina to go to sleep, we talked about the color blue and how it helped with relaxation and rest. I shared that green was a very powerful color for helping them calm down when they were upset. Green is also great for healing when a person is in pain. So we visualized floating on blue clouds while little green aliens flew around and sent them healing green rays. We also talked about yellow being good for thinking and problem solving, pink for love and happiness, purple for confidence, and orange for creativity and fun.

One day, Angelina came home from kindergarten in a terrible mood. She went into the kitchen and began crying and stamping her feet, saying, "I'm not happy!" Within moments, Raphael ran up to her shouting, "Quick, quick! Look at pink! It'll make you happy!" She stopped crying, looked at him, and said, "But I'm wearing pink." Smiling, he said, "The quicker you look at it, the faster you will be happy." Within minutes, Angelina forgot what she was upset about and was laughing.

Healing with Water

Many people are familiar with the work of Dr. Masaru Emoto, who performed a number of experiments observing the physical effect of thoughts, words, prayers, music, energy, and intention on the crystalline structure of water.

Dr. Emoto discovered that water formed into exquisitely complex, shimmering crystal patterns when it was exposed to loving thoughts, words, or feelings and then frozen. Water exposed to negative intentions created disproportionate, often rough and sickly looking patterns, with dull, dark colors.[18]

Since half of the earth and three-quarters of our body is water, those findings shed a lot of light on how our thoughts, words, feelings, vibrations, colors, and behaviors can either have healing or destructive effects on our lives, our planet, and our immune function.

Simon's Story: Charging Water with Color

Simon, eight years old, had very bad asthma. One of the best colors for healing any chest problems, including asthma, is orange. I encouraged Simon to be creative and find a way that he could visualize the orange color whenever he felt out of breath. Simon loved firemen, so every morning, he visualized a fireman with a hose that sprayed orange healing liquid, washing his chest and lungs. I also told his parents to buy an orange glass or cup, put purified water into it, and visualize orange light with healing properties going into the water. Then I told them to place the water in the sun for ten to twenty minutes before giving it to Simon to drink.

Within a month of using this visualization and drinking healing water, Simon felt much better and virtually did not need his inhaler.

This process can be done with any color. After putting some water in a colored glass or cup, you can rub your hands together for about thirty seconds and focus on a particular color. Visualize holding a ray of it in between your hands, think of positive intentions and affirmations, and then hold your hands above the cup for twenty to thirty seconds. Imagine that your positive intention and the ray of light that you visualized are energizing the water.

Boosting Your Child's Confidence

Self-confidence is an important part of wellness, and adults can help guide children toward habits and practices that build self-esteem and social skills, to assist them in childhood and beyond. The greatest gift you can give a child is to be fully present with them, encouraging them to be and to love themselves. You are the most important role model for your children: they learn about life and what they are worth from observing your actions and reactions.

Ten Keys to Boost Self-Esteem in Children

1. Be aware of how you speak to your child. Use encouragement rather than enforcement. Respect and regularly reaffirm your belief in them. Speak to your child about how you would like to be spoken to, and make them feel that what they think counts.

2. Affirm each achievement. Encourage your child to build on his or her progress. Tell your child how clever and intelligent they are and emphasize his or her problem-solving abilities. Then, when another challenge arises, you can remind them that they have faced situations in the past successfully and can do so again.

3. Encourage your child's imagination. Spend time with them, making up stories and adventures together. Allow them to play different roles, so they can learn creative ways of overcoming problems while having fun. This will also demonstrate how to look at situations from different perspectives.

4. Help your child to feel safe and supported. Children need to know that someone is available for them. They need to feel that they are important and valuable human beings, and that, for support, they can easily turn to someone who will listen and believe them.

5. Give your child tasks. For example, encourage them to clean their room. First, demonstrate what you would like done by doing it with them; the next time, ask him or her to do it alone. After they have finished, make sure you check the task and let them know what a wonderful job they have done. If they feel you value their efforts, they will be proud of themselves and likely to do it again.

6. Teach your child to appreciate himself or herself. You can do this by telling them, "You are a lovable child, you have a great imagination, and I'm proud of you." Make sure that you give them regular hugs and kisses so that they feel loved. If they love themselves, they will be more willing to love and see the best in others. If you are tired or annoyed and snap at your child, or push him or her away, apologize as soon as possible. It is important for children to understand that adults make mistakes and are willing to admit to them.

7. Be willing to explain why you want or don't want your child to do something. Just like with an adult, if a child understands the reason, even if he or she doesn't like it, the child will see your purpose and feel less restricted.

8. Honor your child's games. For example, many children enjoy doing the opposite of what they are asked, or saying the opposite of what you are saying. Once you recognize that what they are doing is a game and they are not doing it to upset you, you can join in the fun.

9. Recognize children for who they are as well as what they do. If your child does something that you do not approve of, point out that you do not like this behavior, but you still love him or her and believe they are great.

10. If you have unresolved emotional issues, make sure you work on releasing them so that you don't pass them on to your children. Children are very sensitive to what their parents and other family members are going through, and learn by example. When you let go of an old pattern you have been carrying, you also help to clear this pattern for your children.

Getting children involved in sporting activities also builds self-esteem and social skills. If they don't enjoy sports, encourage them to take a dance class, martial arts workshop, or swimming lessons. Acting and singing classes are also fantastic for developing social skills and compassion, teaching kids to understand each other, be creative, play, connect with their own bodies, and be present. Some teachers also encourage their students to quiet their minds, meditate, breathe deeply, and use visualization skills.

Lilly's Story: Confident Sleeping

Lilly was nine and still sleeping in her parents' bed. Phoebe, Lilly's mum, was at a loss. She had tried therapy and several other treatments for Lilly, which were unsuccessful. Lilly was also putting on weight and being bullied at school. Even though she was an extremely bright young girl, she was losing her confidence.

When I first saw Lilly, I felt it was important to gain her trust by making her feel safe and supported. People often have problems sleeping when they feel insecure and lack trust. Thus, they feel they cannot fall asleep, as they must always be on their guard.

Once I felt Lilly relax, I found out that she loved angels. She had angel cards and played with them often. I asked Lilly to close her eyes and imagine the most beautiful angel she had ever seen helping her to feel safe enough to sleep in her own bed. Lilly visualized the angel and asked her for help. Lilly also told me that her favorite color was purple. As purple is very helpful with sleep disorders, I advised Lilly to visualize beautiful purple and lavender rays of light surrounding her room and bed.

Two months later, Phoebe called to let me know that Lilly was happily sleeping in her own bed. She had also lost weight, was more confident, was able to stand up for herself, and had made more friends.

Processes for Raising Confident Children

Following are two processes that you can practice with your child. I also suggest that you make up specific process for your child based on what I have written. Depending on the age of the child, think of characters that they like and ask your child to visualize them in different situations, helping him or her to feel better. Be creative. If your child is open to it, encourage them to ask angels and fairies for help.

Heal with Color

First find out what issue your child is dealing with. Is it physical, emotional, or mental? Are they being bullied, lacking self-confidence, putting on excess weight, or not eating enough? Then, either pick a color you think will be the most helpful for this problem or ask what their favorite color is. Do not use black, and be very careful not to use too much red, gold, gray, and brown, as they can be overpowering. These colors need to be balanced out with other colors, such as white or orange.

Ask your child to rub his or her hands together for about thirty seconds, making sure he or she rubs every finger. Then ask the child to visualize a particular color. Encourage him or her to make the color as big, shiny, and bright as possible. It is easy to imagine it as a ball or a balloon. Then tell the child to place his or her intention in it. The focus may be the wish to be happier, more confident, do better at school, heal faster, have more friends, and so forth. Ask the child to say the intention out loud and imagine that all those wishes are now going inside the colorful ball of energy.

Tell him or her to breathe in this ball of energy, imagining that the color and the healing intention moves inside the body to release stress, or to make him or her feel stronger and healthier. Ask the child to place his or her hands on the part of the body that feels weak, hurts, or is uncomfortable. Instruct them to keep their hands on this part of the body for a minute or two, breathing in the colorful light.

Form a Positive Intention

Ask your child to repeat: "Divine Healing Intelligence, please help me release any feelings of _____ (ask your child to put in what he or she needs to let go of, like feelings of anger, sadness, fear, stress, and so forth). I am a beautiful, lovable child, and I deserve to feel happy, supported, and cared about. I am capable of great things, and I believe that I can heal quickly and feel better about myself and this situation. Divine Light, please help me feel more confident, happy, and healthy. Thank you."

Ask your child to repeat the word "PEACE" several times, until your child says he or she feels lighter.

Please feel free to adjust this process in a way that suits the child.

Meditate for Better Sleep

Below is a meditation from an audio program, *Color Meditation for Children*, that my children recorded to help other kids use color healing. The process is meant to help a child relax and fall asleep. You can guide your child through this process or make up your own.

Process: The Dolphin with the Blue Crystal

Step 1:

Blue helps you to feel more relaxed and peaceful.

Close your eyes, and take some slow, deep breaths.

Can you think of parts of nature that have the color blue? Think of the ocean, the sky, flowers.

Can you think of any other things or animals that are blue? Imagine floating in cool, clear, blue water.

Step 2:

A dolphin swims close to you and gives you a chance to pat it. You feel happy and playful.

The dolphin opens its mouth and you notice a big blue crystal on its tongue.

The dolphin nods its head to let you know that you can take the crystal.

The dolphin tells you that if you squeeze the crystal once, you will feel very relaxed.

If you squeeze it twice, you will take deep, slow breaths and forget about anything that is upsetting you.

If you squeeze it three times, you will feel so peaceful and calm that you will be able to fall asleep quickly and easily.

Take a moment to think about how many times you would like to squeeze the crystal. Now, imagine doing it.

(If you have a crystal, then you can give it to your child to hold and actually squeeze. Then have your child put it under his or her pillow.)

Feel your body relax.

Imagine breathing in the color blue.

As you breathe out, say to yourself, *I feel peaceful and quiet.*

Allow your thoughts to gently slow down.

Repeat to yourself, *I feel peaceful and calm.*

Feel yourself relaxing more and more, or falling asleep.

Any time you feel a bit worried or upset, imagine squeezing the blue crystal and relaxing deeply.

17

HOW YOU CAN CLEAR
YOUR SPACE AND HOUSE

People often talk about space clearing or house clearing.
What is the benefit of this, and how can I do that for my house?

In the same way people cannot see electricity but still know when it stops flowing in their house once a fuse blows, people can feel when something is energetically out of balance in their living space. For instance, on my first visit to Berlin, I visited some sights with a local friend. As I prefer to let other people navigate in countries I have not been to, I did not know what part of the city we were visiting. Suddenly, I began to feel heavy, anxious, traumatic energy. In fact, I saw images of people screaming, running, and being shot at. When I asked my friend where we were, he told me we were nearing the Berlin Wall. I was not surprised about what I was seeing and feeling, as there had been incredible trauma in that part of Berlin. Since everything on this planet is energetic, it is no wonder that our environment, the earth, and other inanimate objects we build can store energetic information concerning what has occurred there.

Many ancient cultures knew about the benefits of clearing internal and external space, and creating a safe, positive environment from which to blossom and grow.

213

Cleaning Up an Energetic Mess

If your house is unkempt, you will have difficulty concentrating, feeling inspired, and having clarity. The mess will most likely create chaos in your outer and inner life, and until you clean it up, it will make you feel uncomfortable in your environment.

Just as there can be a physical mess in your environment, there can be an energetic mess. Energetic clutter or density occurs when people have negative thoughts, feelings, and experiences that they emit into their own and other people's environments.

You may notice feeling low and heavy, and even experience difficulty breathing after a person who is depressed, drugged, suicidal, sick, or negative has been to your house. You might also notice that you feel uncomfortable every time you visit a particular house, restaurant, building, or outdoor place.

Clearing Entities

There have been many popular television shows and movies that have talked about entities and ghosts. Spirit attachments and exorcisms are discussed in almost every major religion and spiritual teaching around the world.

Over the years, I have had several encounters with beings who have passed over. Often, these beings are lost, have unfinished business, or are looking to go to the light, and they may just need some help.

On many occasions, I have also seen family members who have passed over and need to get a message to a loved one, so they hang around that person.

Although for some people this idea might be inconceivable or uncomfortable, I have witnessed many incredible, almost miraculous changes, both in people and their environments, after I have helped clear entities from their space.

Regularly Clearing Your Space

Clearing your house or business is not a once-a-year process but something that needs to be done regularly. We need to recognize and take care of energetic pollution as much as we take care of the physical pollution in our home. Having a clear, positive, loving environment helps you to relax, attract success, enhance your relationships, and improve your health and sense of well-being.

Sam's Story: Clearing a Spiritual Energy

Sam had a house in a popular suburb that he had not been able to sell for years. When Sam came to see me, he was frustrated and confused about why he could not sell the house. In fact, he desperately needed money to pay off debts and was anxious to sell it, even at a lower price.

Though I rarely do house visits and prefer to teach people the house clearing process, I knew this was special. The moment I walked into Sam's house, I had a sickening feeling. I asked Sam if someone had been sick or died in the house.

Sam told me the house had been his father's, and his father had been extremely ill before he died. His lungs had collapsed as he was dying. I instantly understood why I had difficulty breathing.

When I went upstairs, I felt an invisible wall in front of me, and it took all my energy to go through it. By the time I had walked around the house, I felt drained. Sam told me that the people who came to look at the house often complained of feeling exhausted and unwell as they left.

I spent two hours clearing the dense, heavy energy that had been left in the house, making sure that each room was fresh, clear, and re-energized. I also saw Sam's father, who was still in the house and unhappy about his son's intention to sell. I helped Sam communicate with his father and then guided his father to the light.

When I had completed the clearing, I asked Sam to walk through the house and tell me if he felt any difference. He told me he felt lighter, joyous, and at ease. I also encouraged him to bring some flowers, colorful objects, or potted plants to restore some life to the house.

A week later, I received a phone call from an excited Sam. He said that not only had he sold his house and gotten a fantastic price, but the new owners could not stop saying how fresh and clear the house felt. He said that when they came downstairs, they told him the house was exactly what they were looking for, as they felt energized and at peace in it. Sam was amazed that they did not even try to bargain.

Piotr's Story: Clearing His Shop

Another powerful space-clearing experience occurred with Piotr, my twin soul and one of my closest friends. I had just begun teaching in Paris, and every day, as I walked toward the center, I passed his couture boutique. Since I have a deep love of beautiful clothes, I looked at Piotr's designs with awe. The dresses in his windows were stunning. I was so in love with his creations that I promised myself that, one day, I would own a beautiful dress made by him.

However, I felt very uncomfortable about entering his shop. It was couture, and to go in, you needed an appointment. One day, while sitting with the owner of a spiritual shop in Paris, I had a strong compulsion to go into Piotr's shop. I tried to resist the feeling, but it seemed impossible. In fact, I felt like an angel was whispering in my ear, "Go into the shop, go into the shop, go into the shop!" Before I knew it, I felt someone turn my head toward the shop owner and heard myself telling her that I was going to Piotr's shop.

Surprised, she said, "Don't talk to him about anything spiritual, as he doesn't believe in this stuff."

I told her that it was not a problem, as I could talk about clothes as much as I could talk about anything spiritual.

When I got the courage to go into the shop, Piotr and I clicked instantly. I felt a deep connection to him and an ease that completely surprised me. After some friendly chatter, Piotr asked me what work I did. Without hesitation, I said, "Healing."

He looked at me strangely before muttering, "I am not sick, so I do not need healing."

I answered, "Healing is not just for pain and sickness. And if you think you don't need it, then you are either deluded or do not understand healing." He seemed taken aback but interested.

I decided to ask him if he had many clients. I knew that he had leased the shop and started the business about three months previously. He said, "Why do you ask?" I told him that I did not know what had occurred in the shop before he leased it, but the energy was atrocious. I could see and feel people screaming, getting angry, and feeling upset. I told him that if he did have clients, it would be because of his amazing ability to inspire them. Whenever his clients entered the shop, those heavy energies were most likely pushing them out the door.

Piotr asked me if and when I could help clear his shop and also give him a healing session. We agreed on the next day. When I next saw the owner of the spiritual shop, she was amazed that Piotr wanted a healing session. She was even more astonished when I told her what I had seen in his shop. She shared that, before Piotr moved in, it was a shop that sold kitchens. The man who owned it was a crook and a liar. She told me that people often came into the shop and screamed at the owner for deceiving them and taking their money.

The next day, I went to Piotr's shop and cleared the heavy energy. In a few days, his business increased dramatically. He also realized healing is a way of life, rather than just a way to relieve pain. Since then, he has participated in many of my workshops, and assisted me at conferences and events.

Process for Clearing Space

This is a shortened yet effective version of an in-depth process that I teach in Visionary Intuitive Healing® seminars. It is advisable that you do a process for protecting yourself before you do this clearing (see page 114). You must do the space-clearing process separately for every room.

Walk into a room that you would like to clear. Close your eyes and imagine surrounding the room with soft blue light. Call on Divine Healing Intelligence.

Hold your left hand near the upper part of your chest, with your palm facing away from you, as if you are greeting someone. All your fingers should be extended upward. Raise your right hand with your elbow facing out. Bend your middle and ring finger and place your thumb just below the nail of your ring finger. Keep your index finger and little finger extended. Hold your right hand in front of your solar plexus.

Say the following statement out loud or to yourself: "I ask the Divine Source to cleanse this room of all density; energetic, emotional, and mental toxicity; negativity; fear; pain; and dis-ease. Please lovingly return any spirits or beings who have been stuck here to their rightful place. Please cleanse and return any fragments of energy that have been left in this room to their rightful owners. Divine Source, dissipate all negative energy and transform it into light. Fill this space with love, lightness, joy, and clarity, so that anyone who enters this room feels at ease and at peace. Allow anyone who enters this space to reconnect with their wisdom, and assist them to come into alignment with who they really are. Thank you."

Repeat the word "CLEAR" several times, until you feel lighter.

Hold your hand positions for another thirty to sixty minutes, or until you feel that the room has become lighter. Then visualize a rainbow light surrounding the room.

218

18

How You Can Create More Money and Success in Your Life

I want to be successful and have an abundance of money.
However, I feel really uncomfortable with having money.
In fact, whenever I have it, I find a way to give it away quickly or lose it.
What can I do?

Apowerful way to move toward success is to examine your beliefs and attitudes about money and abundance. What kinds of clichés have you internalized? Have you been taught that money doesn't grow on trees, is hard to get, and that rich people are crooks?

I have often asked my workshop participants to write down their beliefs about money for three minutes, without stopping. I then inquire: "Did you know you believe all this? Do you think a person who believes this could attract money easily?" This opens a lively discussion on what kind of consistent thoughts, feelings, and actions create abundance.

When I interviewed Suze Orman, two-time Emmy Award–winning television host, *New York Times* bestselling author, and expert on personal finance, she said, "I believe with all my heart that your thoughts create your destiny. You have to be very, very careful about what you think, because what you think, you eventually say; words become your actions, your actions become your habits, and your habits become your destiny. So you might think and say, 'I want to be financially free' but take absolutely no actions to make that become a reality. True change happens when your thoughts, your words, and your actions are one."[19]

We do not have to live our lives with the limiting beliefs of our ancestors. If this is not the time to allow more prosperity in, then when is it? Rather than having money control your life, allow yourself to learn how to become empowered with it.

It is important to recognize that we have the ability to manifest great things into our lives, as well as challenging and unpleasant experiences. It is also interesting to note that it actually takes more energy to manifest what we don't want than what we do. When you manifest what you don't want, you weaken your attractor field; on the other hand, when you manifest what you desire, you feel pleasure and increase your energy.

A great affirmation to repeat is *I manifest abundance with ease, grace, and joy.*

Becoming Friendly with Money

The first step you need to take in creating wealth is to become friendly with money. Ask yourself how much money you would be comfortable having in your wallet. How much money would you love to have in your wallet? If you can, carry that amount with you for at least thirty days. Do not spend it. However, note if you feel differently having a large amount of money on you. The more you feel good, powerful, and abundant having a lot of money, the more likely you are to attract it.

I once met a successful businessman who shared with me that he carries at least $10,000 in his wallet because he feels good having a lot of money at his disposal, even if he doesn't spend it. I asked how he would feel if he lost it, to which he replied that he believes he would get it back within twenty-four hours.

Letting Go of Your Fears of Poverty

As a child, I spent my first nine years in Russia, where poverty consciousness was rife, and people considered money to be something only crooks had. I realized how affected I had been when I examined my beliefs about lack and not having enough, especially when I worried incessantly about how I would pay my bills.

The threat of survival stops a lot of people, not only from living their dreams but from asking themselves what they really want. It's like they are afraid to find out, in case it's something interesting and creative that may require them to take risks or start from scratch. Many people also put a lot of their attention on limitations and not having enough, rather than on cocreation and the idea that there is more than enough.

What most people don't realize is that success takes time, persistence, passion, trust, belief, and support. Your desire to create has to emanate from you and then inspire others to come on board.

When I spent time with Robert Kiyosaki, a famous financial educator and bestselling author of *Rich Dad, Poor Dad*, he shared, "I've been broke three times. I was born into a poor family and lost two companies. I understand what it feels like to be poor. Some people say, 'I don't have money; that's why I can't become rich,' and I like to say, 'I became rich because I didn't have any money—because I had to become rich. I used adversity to become rich.'"[20]

In order to increase my prosperity, I began affirming and noticing everything I already had. I would walk into a park and think: *Wow, how fortunate am I to be able to sit in this beautiful park and smell the flowers.* Each day, I would take time to recognize how abundant I was, to focus on gratitude, and to tell myself: *There is more where this came from.*

I also decided to become friends with money, so every day, I looked at a twenty-, fifty-, or hundred-dollar bill and told it that I loved it. Whenever I paid for anything, I blessed the money and asked that it return to me ten times. The more I practiced, the more comfortable I became with money—and it began to multiply. Rather than seeing money as something physical that created stress, I began to view it as energy that allowed freedom of choice.

Believing in a Hundredfold Return

Emily was a workshop participant who wanted to expand her manifestation abilities. In a particular exercise, Emily gave a twenty-dollar bill to another participant, blessed it, closed her eyes, relaxed, and asked the money to return to her a hundredfold within one week. Emily had no idea where the money would come from, but she felt confident that it would. She could imagine and feel it coming, and welcomed it.

The following week, Emily received $2,000 from a family member who had never given her money previously.

This is a little experiment that I have done in several workshops, and the results are always astounding.

I once did it in Mexico, where a woman gave over a $1,000 to another participant. I saw her six months later, and she shared that, within a few months of that experiment, her business increased by 70 percent and she multiplied her money manyfold.

This experiment has demonstrated time and time again how our focus, energy, feelings, and thoughts about money influence where and how it manifests in our lives.

Amanda's Story: Clarity and Consistency

Amanda attended my workshop because she wanted to learn how to be more grounded and to manifest greater things. A single mother of two small children, she needed a job. I asked Amanda to tell me about the kind of job she desired. She told me she wanted to work for a company that cared about the environment and children. She had her heart set on a sales position with all the perks of having a company car, good salary, computer, flexible hours, occasional travel, and fun. She needed this job within a month.

We looked at Amanda's beliefs about finding a job and worked on letting go of limiting ideas, fears, and self-sabotage. Amanda was on the right track: she had a clear intention of what she wanted and was willing to go after it. Amanda also focused on creating a feeling that she had already achieved her goal. Now, she just needed to have trust and be open to Divine Inspiration.

That month, Amanda attended a few interviews and received some offers. However, none of the jobs fit her requirements. She was desperate, as time and money were running out. Fortunately, Amanda had made a promise to herself that she was not going to settle and accept second best. She had done it too many times, and this time was going to be different.

A week before her one-month deadline, Amanda was on her way home from yet another disappointing interview when she asked herself, "What would be the best company for me to work for?" Suddenly, the name of a company entered her mind. *It would be great to work for them*, she thought. *I'll call the company as soon as I get home.* But her intuition told her, "Call now!"

Amanda stopped by the side of the road, found the company's number, and called. To her amazement, the owner picked up the phone and told her she had just spoken to her partners about expanding and employing a new salesperson.

They set up a meeting and Amanda got her dream job.

Aligning with Our Greatest Good

Wealthy people I have spent time with have often told me they believe they can make money no matter where they are. Their secret is that they do what they love with a fiery passion, and they completely focus on prosperity.

Part of creating a life of prosperity is knowing what you love and going for it. Too often, people have an intention of something they would like to create, then settle for less because it is easier.

I believe that when we align ourselves with our greatest good, and open our hearts to receive it, it appears. Often, we cannot predict how something will happen; we just need to trust and take steps toward it. Synchronicity is a message from the universe that tells us we are on the right track.

In order for you to become truly successful, your heart must be completely invested in your dreams. Although it is possible to achieve a high level of success without having your heart in it, the level of satisfaction is limited. You are likely to feel empty, unfulfilled, and lose the money you accumulate.

Robert Kiyosaki says, "I only do what I love and invest in what I love. I would never do something just for money."[21]

Cocreating Your Desires

The clearer your chakras are, the faster your energy flows, bringing what you dream of—or something better—into your life. When I talk about cocreation, I see it as you creating your desires hand in hand with your soul and Divine Guidance. The experience feels organic, easy, and enjoyable. During challenging times, your wisdom and intuition help you access creative solutions. A question I often ask Divine Intelligence is "How does this get better?" Then I focus on how things can improve, rather than on why they are not working.

There are many other steps that can help you to become successful. These include clarifying and writing your goals, working with mentors, creating a vision board, visualizing your goals manifesting, taking daily action steps, and creating a great team of people who can support you.

Linking Success

In order to increase your productivity and achievement, link your present skills to what you would love to do. For example, you may have studied accounting and are good with numbers, but you want to do something creative. Instead of disregarding accounting and thinking that it was a waste of time, recognize how accounting could help you in the future. You may want to set up your own business, and knowing how to work with numbers can help you make your business flourish.

You may consider all the different things you do and enjoy to be random and disconnected. If you take time to link these, however, you may be pleasantly surprised at how they fit into your life and how they could bring all kinds of possibilities. Opportunities may not come instantly but appear in time, in unexpected ways.

You can also apply this principle by linking your daily tasks to your practice of certain manifestation techniques I have described in this chapter. For example, you may already do the dishes once or twice daily. Instead of washing them in an irritated or dazed way, focus on being present: relax your muscles; take slow, deep breaths; repeat affirmations; clarify your intentions; and visualize more money or abundance coming into your life.

Tim's Story: Link to the Life You Love

Tim worked in a communication company, but his background was in science. When I met Tim, he was unhappy and confused about what he wanted to do. I asked him what his passion was, and he replied, "Writing." He particularly loved creating empowering poetry. He was also excited about helping people. However, he could not see how those things could be linked. I told him that his background in science could help him understand the human body better, while working in communication could help him talk to people. His passion for writing could be used to write articles about the subjects he loved. I also encouraged him to start a blog where he could share his poetry.

In time, Tim quit his job, assisted me in different workshops, and saw clients for healing. During certain seminars, he read his poetry, which inspired people and gave him confidence. Tim now sees how everything he did in the past supports him in living the life he loves.

My Story: Success, Step by Step

When I was growing up, I wanted to be an actress and a writer. Through attending acting classes, I learned about my emotions, my thoughts, and how other people feel and think. I discovered how to connect to my intuition and follow it. I also felt that, by following my passion and having an open heart, I would meet people who would love, guide, and support me. When I met Paul, he helped me explore different types of healing modalities.

I linked my love of writing with my enthusiasm for healing, and interviewed many successful and wise people. I was then able to sell my articles to magazines, which made me feel empowered as a journalist. Once I'd decided that I wanted a private practice and to work with clients, I made agreements with the editors of various magazines I wrote for to exchange my articles for advertising. This brought me lots of clients.

I then decided to link my love of communication and sharing with my desire to see people become self-empowered and heal: I began to teach. As I continued to explore what brought me joy and happiness, I realized that I wanted to travel to many different countries, experience new cultures, and make deep and profound friendships.

My desire to be of service led to travel, and I began to receive invitations to speak and lead workshops in different countries. My curiosity about various cultures helped me develop deep friendships and gave me insights into new ways of living life. The more experiences I had, the more inspired I was to return to my love of writing, sharing my insights with people all over the world.

Manifesting Prosperity with Chakras

I have mentioned the power of understanding and working with the chakra system several times throughout this book. This section is an exploration of how cocreation of success works with and through the chakra system.

The process begins at the ninth chakra, which is your soul chakra. This is where you find the seeds of inspiration for your life purpose. When these seeds are stimulated, the energy of creation moves in to the eighth chakra, your Akashic Records chakra. At this level, your soul tunes into any past beliefs or skills that will help you succeed. This is known as talent.

If clear, your seventh chakra (or crown chakra) can help you to connect with your Divinity, expand your vision, and embrace your gifts. As you develop your dreams, the sixth chakra, known as the third-eye chakra, helps you clarify your ideas. This is where you visualize future possibilities and potential achievements.

The fifth chakra, the throat chakra, helps you communicate your goals and desires to others. However, until you become extremely confident with the cocreation process, it is very important to share your ideas only with people who will understand and support you, thus increasing the power of your vision.

The fourth chakra, also known as the heart chakra, requires you to work with your heart. If your heart is open, loving, and passionate, your capacity to attract supportive people and extraordinary opportunities intensifies.

The last three chakras are vital to manifesting your goals into physical reality. The third chakra, or solar plexus chakra, requires you to invest time, money, energy, and other valuable resources into your idea.

The second chakra—the sacral chakra—requires you to take deliberate steps toward making your dreams a reality. The more clear and determined you are, understanding your potential challenges and blessings, the more chances you have to manifest your dreams on a larger scale. The sacral chakra is the last place where you can abort your goals. However, stopping at this point can contribute to serious emotional and physical issues in your body. The most common are cysts in the reproductive area for women and prostate problems for men.

In the first chakra, also known as the root chakra, your ideas are no longer just your own. In order to achieve great things, you need support. This chakra sends powerful vibrations into the world, which in turn attracts people, finances, and opportunities to make your vision a reality.

Expanding Your Nervous System to Handle Abundance

During a time when I was meeting and often doing healing sessions on well-known authors, actors, and entertainers, I discovered that the more successful the person, the more expanded his or her nervous system looked—like the nervous system was magnified outside the body. Later, I realized that I was observing their etheric bodies, which appeared huge. I understood that this reflected the amount of opportunities, money, and recognition these enormously successful people were able to embrace.

I then paid attention to people who struggled with money. I noticed that their nervous systems seemed smaller, tighter, and stuck. I began working with these people on expanding their nervous systems, and holding more abundance and possibility. Invariably, I received amazing feedback about more money, success, and incredible opportunities coming into their lives.

Embracing Failure and Remaining Persistent

Even if you fail while trying to do what you really want to do, at least you gave it a go. Failure means that the path you took did not work at that time, so your opportunity is to be creative and find a different way to do what you love and believe in. Often, the learning experience of failure is invaluable in making your dreams a great success. Many of the world's most successful people made lots of mistakes, lost large amounts of money, and failed at one or more businesses before they reached a high level of wealth and accomplishment. So, while failure is the end of a dream for some, for others, it is a stepping-stone to success.

Many people allow their fear of failure and rejection to stop them from going on an extraordinary journey. However, everyone I have ever met, interviewed, or read about who has achieved or experienced an amazing life has had the courage to face fear in order to live their dreams.

- Richard Bach's 10,000-word story about a soaring seagull, *Jonathan Livingston Seagull*, was rejected by eighteen publishers until one brave person (at a publishing house that had previously rejected the book) read the manuscript and commited to printing the book no matter what anyone else said. By 1975, the book sold seven million copies in the United States alone.
- Robert Kiyosaki originally self-published his books because everybody turned him down. His books now have combined sales of over twenty-six million copies.
- Susan Jeffers, author of *Feel the Fear and Do It Anyway*, received a letter from a publisher that read, "If Princess Diana flogged this book naked on a horse, no one would read it." *Feel the Fear and Do It Anyway* became an international bestseller.

Processes for Creating a Positive Relationship with Money

Here are five powerful exercises to help you accelerate your prosperity. I highly recommend that you practice them regularly. Work daily with the process for examining and deleting your beliefs, as well as the process for expanding your nervous system, as both are very powerful in creating fast and lasting changes.

Practice Holding Money

Hold some money in your hands. Ask yourself how you feel about it. Are you holding a little bit of money or a lot of money? Do you feel comfortable or uncomfortable? How much money do you feel comfortable having in your wallet, in your bank account, in your home? Are you comfortable with just a little or a lot? Every day, practice holding more money than you are used to, increasing your comfort levels.

Examine Your Beliefs

Let's examine some of your beliefs. When you focus on creating money, you need to understand what deeply ingrained beliefs you may carry. Often, those beliefs come from your parents and your childhood. Do you believe that money is bad, not spiritual, hard to get? Do you tell yourself that there is not enough money? Do you ever say that you don't care about money, judge it, and judge people who have it? Do you feel controlled by money? Do you feel limited and tell others you would be happy if you had just enough to pay your bills?

For five minutes, write down as many negative beliefs about money as you can think of, without stopping. Once you have done that, look at each one and do the simple deleting process written below.

Say: "Divine Healing Intelligence, please help me delete, delete, delete my limiting beliefs about money, such as _____ (put in a belief), as well as all points of view and positive and negative charge. Thank you."

Repeat the word "CLEAR" several times, until you feel lighter.

Positive and Negative Charge

Part of the healing statement is to release positive and negative charges. When we have a charge on someone or something, we often react strongly to that person, event, or experience. A negative charge could be based on a strong negative feeling like anger, hate, fear, jealousy, and so on. A positive charge could be based on a strong need, expectation, feeling of impatience, and so on.

For instance, you may have just gotten a new job and feel over the moon about it. You may have ideas and expectations about what you are going to do and learn in this new job. Then you discover that the reality at work is very different from what you had hoped. Thus, you become frustrated and depressed, and the positive charge turns negative. Ideally, we want to release all charges and allow Divinity, synchronicity, and well-being to flow into our lives.

To help with this, my healing processes are always followed by the word "CLEAR," as a reminder to clear all density, pain, stress, and limitation out of your mind, body, emotions, and vibration. When you repeat the word "CLEAR," imagine a broom or a vacuum cleaner clearing any mess out of your system, or clearing a pathway for you to experience wonderful things in your life. Repeat the word several times until you can tell something has cleared, indicated by your feeling lighter, more at ease, freer, tingly, or more open to new possibilities.

I have also discovered that when you repeat the word "CLEAR" often, taking a moment to visualize until you feel the clutter disappear, you will start having more clarity in your life, your memory will improve, and you will able to manifest more of the things you desire. Your body will also work better because each time you say "CLEAR," your nervous system will begin to clear any stuckness you have, improving the communication between your mind and body. Some people see results from these exercises immediately, but if you do not, remember that just as it can take time for disease to develop, sometimes it also takes time to find health and wellness again.

Visualize an Abundant Childhood

Think about what you felt toward money when you were a child. If your family was poor or struggled with money, you may still carry these memories in your mind. A meditation you can do: Imagine yourself as a child, except this time, you have the things you always wanted but were unable to have before. Picture what it would have been like if your family had had plenty of money, and you were able to enjoy it. Allow yourself to feel good about having money. Then visualize yourself growing up with a lot of money and all the opportunities that money provides. The intention is to build a feeling of abundance and change ingrained childhood patterns.

See Yourself and Others as Abundant

For the next month, think of your friends and the people you meet as having an abundance of money. This way, you will reprogram your subconscious mind from lack to plenty. Practice seeing them as abundant every time you think of, speak to, or see them.

Look at money every day and tell it that you like it, or even that you love it. The better you feel about money, the more likely it will come into your life. Treat it like you would treat a good friend. Bless your money every time you pay someone or pay your bills, and ask that it return to you tenfold. Then imagine receiving it.

Write down and clarify your goals and dreams. Take daily steps toward making these a reality; it does not matter how big or small the step. The important part is for you to be consistent.

Expand Your Nervous System

Rub your hands together vigorously, then hold them apart about two to four inches. You should feel a tingling sensation. Imagine holding a big ball of green light between your hands. Focus on receiving more money, abundance, and fantastic opportunities than you have ever experienced. Imagine that the energetic potential of all these opportunities are now being infused into this green ball of energy. Focus on feeling joyful at the possibility of receiving these great things. The better you feel when you are focused on manifesting, the faster it happens.

Allow that green ball of energy to grow.

Place your hands on your mid-back and breathe in. Visualize your whole nervous system expanding and aligning to your dreams as it is flooded with the powerful green rays of light. Imagine receiving what you have asked for. Focus on embracing it with your whole being. Give yourself permission to own and enjoy it. Be grateful that you can manifest your dreams. The more real it feels, the faster you will receive it.

Give yourself permission to be receptive to intuitive and Divine Guidance, and to take the necessary steps toward your goal.

Invoke Success

Say the following statement out loud or to yourself: "I accept my good on all levels: mental, emotional, energetic, spiritual, and physical. I now open my mind, heart, and soul to receive intuitive direction and Divine Guidance about my dreams. I now choose to align myself with all the richness of life, which is for my highest good. I attract success and wonderful opportunities for me. Thank you."

Repeat the word "AMPLIFY" several times, until you feel lighter.

The reason to repeat Amplify is so that you can strengthen the process and make your prosperity grow!

PART IV

LETTING GO

The last part of this book is about taking off and letting go. As you let go of excess emotional, physical, and energetic weight, you become lighter and have the capacity to make new, empowered choices—choices that help you take off and become more successful in your life.

When your point of view about yourself and your life changes, your capacity to become a present, full participant of your life dramatically increases. Thus, you become softer, and more loving and accepting of yourself. When you let go of something in your life, whether it is an old belief, your weight, emotional discontent, a relationship, a house, a country, or a way of life, you have the possibility of welcoming new people, opportunities, love, joy, growth, compassion, and soulfulness into your daily experience.

Letting go is an important and often difficult part of maturing and moving forward.

19

HOW YOU CAN LOVE YOUR BODY AND ATTAIN YOUR IDEAL WEIGHT

*I have struggled with my weight for many years, trying every diet under the sun, but
nothing seems to work. My weight issue is highly emotional;
it is possible it goes back to my childhood. I have never felt happy in my body and
have always judged it. I am ready to love my body and let go of any excess weight.
Can you please share some of your insights about weight loss?*

Obesity is one of the biggest health problems facing the world today. Stress, fast
food, financial instability, lack of exercise, and an unhealthy lifestyle have contrib-
uted to weight gain. Although diet and exercise are vital in order to maintain a healthy
body, unresolved emotions and deeply ingrained negative thought patterns can play a
huge role in holding on to unnecessary weight.

Stop Substituting Food for Love

Many people use food as a substitute for love, communication, and support, and as a
way to stuff down their feelings. Your body can also hold on to weight when it feels
under threat and in need of protection. Unconsciously, you may carry a belief that the
bigger you are, the stronger you will be, and that no one will be able to hurt you. More
than ever before, people are experiencing the pressure to rise to the top of their professions, make substantial incomes, travel, have stable family lives, spend time with their
children, and (in other words) be superhuman.

Often, this leaves little time for us to connect to our bodies, eat consciously, deal with challenging issues, and heal painful emotions.

Recognizing Your Worth

Girls and boys, younger than ever before, are developing eating disorders because they are sold a particular image of beauty. Weight problems typically begin early, with feelings of not being good enough, self-judgment, and a deep need for love and approval.

When people are abused, taken advantage of, or traumatized, they can develop a negative self-image and punish themselves by eating unhealthy food and putting on weight. Then they feel guilty and beat themselves up for being heavy, beginning a never-ending cycle of feeling fat, bad, and like a failure. They often see themselves as ugly, overweight, and worthless.

Recognizing your beauty, Divinity, and worth can help you to take care of yourself, make better choices, heal, and lose weight. Connecting to your body can be very confrontational, however, as it will show you what you believe about yourself, the hurts you hold on to, and how you treat yourself.

In order to change, make the decision that you are lovable and have the courage to make new choices. Taking care of yourself both internally and externally can help you feel good about yourself, increase your self-confidence, and open doors to incredible opportunities, relationships, friendships, jobs, and most important, contentment.

Laura's Story: Owning Her Beauty

Laura had been obese for more than fifteen years. When I tuned in to her, I knew that a traumatic experience had caused her to gain weight. Laura recalled that when she was going through her divorce, she dressed up and went with friends to a sporting event. A man passed her and whistled. At that moment, Laura heard her soon-to-be ex-husband, who also happened to be at the event, make a crude and painful comment.

Laura was so humiliated that she instantly closed up, and disowned her attractiveness and desirability. Within a few months, she had gained an enormous amount of weight. Repulsed by what had happened, she did all she could to appear unattractive to men, so that she would never again invite that kind of sexual attention.

It took a substantial amount of time for Laura to forgive her ex-husband and move forward. She is still in the process of embracing her beauty and sensuality.

I encouraged Laura to change her attitude toward her body and herself, and discover how she could see and treat herself differently. Laura became softer and more loving in her attitude to her body. She also worked on feeling more comfortable with men.

Karen's Story: Losing the Weight of a Traumatic Experience

Karen contacted me because, no matter what she did, she simply could not lose weight. She'd gained excess weight in her childhood and developed a lifelong battle with the bulge.

When I tuned in to Karen, I saw that as a young girl she had been very skinny. I knew something serious happened to her when she was younger, as images of hospitalization flashed through my mind. I had a feeling that Karen had almost died. I saw her soul float out of her body, which was surrounded by people who were commenting that she looked so thin and fragile that they did not think that she would make it.

Upon hearing these words, Karen had made a subconscious decision to put on weight so that she could be strong and healthy, and not end up on the verge of death. She had observed the pain that it caused her family and felt guilty. She also felt an immense responsibility and desire to make her family happy. Since this was a life-and-death situation, Karen's vow to hold on to her weight was strong.

Karen was astonished to discover that this experience was stopping her from shedding the weight. Once she recognized what had happened, she worked with her inner child, creating a new set of choices. Within a short period of time, her weight began to drop, as she no longer needed to protect this part of her.

She also created a new, healthy relationship with food, no longer starving herself and then putting on weight.

Learning to Listen to Your Body

It is important to become friendly with your body and listen to it. Before you eat, ask yourself: *Am I hungry? Or do I want to put food into my mouth because I'm feeling an emotion I'm not comfortable with? Am I eating out of habit, or am I listening to my body?* If you are hungry, take a few moments to check in with your body: what would be the healthiest, most nourishing food that you could eat?

Eat slowly, chew, and taste every mouthful. Enjoy the experience. Stop when your body has had enough, rather than stuffing it.

Many people think they are hungry when, in reality, they are actually thirsty or dehydrated. Check in with yourself before you eat, to see if it is actually water that would satisfy you.

The Minnesota Starvation Experiment, conducted at the University of Minnesota, was a clinical study to determine the physiological and psychological effects of strict and prolonged semi-starvation. Researchers discovered that prolonged dietary restriction produced severe emotional distress and depression; social withdrawal and isolation; decline in concentration, comprehension, and decision making; self-mutilation; and obsessive behavior around food.[22]

Even after the experiment had concluded and people could eat whatever they desired, they were completely preoccupied with food. In fact, many ate up to eight times as much food as they had before the experiment.

Stewart's Story: Overcoming a Vicious Cycle

Stewart put on a lot of weight from the stress of moving to a new country. He had to learn English, find a job, and make new friends. He did not speak English well, so the jobs that he was offered were menial. This made Stewart feel depressed, as he had been well paid in his home country. He also had difficulty making friends and integrating into the new culture.

Stewart felt angry, rejected, hopeless. In his eyes, he was a failure, so when he wanted to feel better, he ate chocolate, sweets, and cake. When he was trying to punish himself, he ate ice cream, chips, and cake. It was a vicious cycle: he would gorge, become disgusted, and fast for weeks. Then after a certain period of deprivation, he binged for a week and put on more weight than he'd lost.

I encouraged Stewart to connect to his strongest emotion; he described it as hopelessness and anger. I asked him to visualize his anger and hopelessness as if it were a person and communicate with it. Stewart saw this aspect as a huge bomb that was about to erupt. As he talked to and listened to this part of himself, tears rolled down his face.

Stewart realized that he had to stop putting unrealistic expectations on himself and become gentler.

I asked Stewart if he knew anybody who was health conscious and enjoyed exercise. He told me that he had recently met a man who loved bike riding and going to the gym. I encouraged Stewart to reach out to him and suggested they exercise together.

I saw Stewart three months later and hardly recognized him. He had lost forty-five pounds, and looked healthy and muscular. He told me that he was training at the gym with his new friend five to six times a week, eating healthy, and feeling better than ever. His English had also improved, and he had been offered a new job that he liked.

Stewart had stopped channeling all his energy into being miserable and started focusing on what he wanted to experience in his life, then taking appropriate action to achieve it.

Developing a Life of Wellness

The main idea is to not only lose weight but to also develop a healthy lifestyle. Here are some tips to get you started.

Drink a glass of water with half of a squeezed lemon when you wake up.

Eat organic food when possible.

Eat a meal within thirty minutes of waking up.

Drink a glass of water before a meal.

Smell your favorite fragrance, some flowers, or essential oils before you eat, as smell can lessen hunger.

Listen to slow, restful music during a meal to encourage you to eat slower and more consciously, and to enjoy your food more. Thus, you may be satisfied with less.

Cut down on the amount of alcohol you drink.

When you feel like snacking, eat a handful of mixed, unsalted nuts or a piece of fruit, instead of sweets.

Press an acupressure "gum point" in the middle of your top lip. Hold it for about ninety seconds, then drink some water. (If you constantly crave snacks, acupressure can help to lower your appetite.)

Stop eating when you are no longer hungry, even if there is still food on your plate.

Eat meals that are colorful, as ingesting certain colors can help you heal.

Eat at regular times.

Cook at home as much as possible.

Cook with coconut and sesame oils, as many other oils become rancid and turn into a carcinogen when you introduce high heat.

Cut down on fried food.

Throw out all the junk food in your cupboards and only buy healthy food. If the junk food isn't there, you can't be tempted.

Exercise four to five times a week, and make it fun and full of variety.

Work on your emotions daily by doing the exercise from the section "Process for Releasing Emotions" on page 96.

Carry a bottle of water with you wherever you go, and drink this rather than soda and other sugary drinks.

Reduce the amount of fat, sugar, and salt in your diet.

Add exercises like lunges, single-leg raises, and squats to the exercises you do.

Visualize yourself reaching your ideal weight.

Go to this link to learn more about the food and beverages that will help you to stay healthy, prevent cancer and heart disease, burn fat, and energize you.
http://innasegal.com/the-secret-of-life-wellness-downloads/healthy-foods-and-beverages

Dianne's Story: An Amazing Physical Transformation

Dianne lost weight and baffled many practitioners in the medical community with her physical transformation. The following is Dianne's story in her own words:

"My journey with weight started many years ago. As a young woman, my weight was considered average. During my adolescent development, I began attracting a lot of attention from older males in my extended family, who began to make sexual advances toward me. I didn't realize the effect this unwanted attention would have on me in the future.

"My parents put me down. No matter what I did or how hard I tried, I was never good enough for them. My weight increased dramatically when my mum pressured me to terminate a pregnancy because I was not married. I felt like I was a huge disappointment to my parents.

"After that, I had two children and was diagnosed as a type 2 diabetic.

"Twelve months after the birth of my youngest daughter, I was given Inna's book, *The Secret Language of Your Body*. Then I attended her workshop, when I was at my heaviest. On the second day of the workshop, I started to feel different. I also noticed that I looked and felt lighter. This was the beginning of my weight-loss journey. Since then, I have attended several Visionary Intuitive Healing® workshops, have worked with Inna's audio programs (in particular *Lose Weight Fast*), and have lost more than forty-five pounds.

"In the last eighteen months, I have released a lot of emotional issues, been taken off blood pressure and depression medication, and have reduced my diabetes medication. I have been told by doctors that this is unheard of in the medical profession.

"In the middle of last year, my doctor advised that I go on cholesterol medication but he agreed to give me six months to reduce my levels without medication. With the help of Inna's workshops, audio programs, exercise, and further dietary changes, within three months, I no longer required any medication.

"I have also quit my stressful job that I had been in for twenty-two years and started my own business. I also have begun enjoying regular exercise and I am now relaxed and much happier."

Process for Losing Weight

The following is one of the processes that Dianne and many others have used to help with weight loss. You need a red blanket and two cups, one red and one white. Fill both cups with water to enhance the process.

Relax

Choose a quiet place where you can make yourself comfortable. Sit on a chair or lie down in a relaxed position. If possible, cover yourself with the red blanket. Allow your eyes to close naturally as you become aware of the inflow and outflow of each breath.

Now that you are comfortable, take a deep breath through your nose, and imagine your breath flowing through your entire body like a wave. As you exhale, bring your attention back to your head. Feel yourself beginning to relax.

Release Negative Thoughts and Feelings

Become aware of your thoughts and feelings about yourself and your weight. Do you feel guilt, anger, fear, or frustration? Do you feel insecure and doubtful about your ability to lose weight quickly and easily?

If you have any of these feelings or others you would like to release, repeat: "I ask the Divine Healing Intelligence of my body to delete, delete, delete all doubts. Melt away all anger, fear, guilt, insecurity, self-doubt, and negativity about my ability to lose weight and to keep it off."

Repeat the word "RELEASE" several times, until you feel lighter, in order to let go of the limiting belief.

Visualize Dissolving Extra Weight

Sense or picture that you are holding a vacuum cleaner. Take this vacuum cleaner and imagine sucking out all the heaviness and density you don't need from your body. Focus especially on the areas of your body that carry extra weight. Imagine pouring bright red energy through your body, allowing it to flow to the parts that are stuck and have been unable to let go of any unnecessary weight. Observe how the weight dissolves. See and feel this taking place.

Repeat the phrase three times: "Divine Healing Intelligence of my body, install, install, install my body's ability to burn fat quickly and easily."

Allow the following statement to penetrate deeply into your subconscious mind: *My body now knows how to burn fat quickly and easily.*

Drink Some Water

To make the process even more powerful, sit up and drink some water from the red cup or glass. If you don't have a red glass, imagine drinking red liquid.

243

Lie down, relax even further, and focus on how this red liquid activates your metabolism and the fat-burning abilities of your body. Your metabolism will speed up to the most appropriate level for you to maintain a healthy, strong, fit body.

Now sit up and drink some water from the white glass, or imagine doing so. Follow the clear liquid as it moves through your body, cleansing, balancing, and regenerating it.

Tap Your Fingers

Using the fingers of both hands, gently tap your forehead while repeating four times: "I now attain my perfect weight." The tapping action will help your body to remember the statement. Then tap your fingers under your eyes, repeating the above statement four times. Finally, tap your fingers around your chest/heart area while taking deep, slow breaths. Repeat the same statement four times. This helps you to release stagnation and instill your intention to lose weight.

Visualize Merging with Your Perfect Self

Imagine being your perfect weight. How do you look? How do you feel? What do you do? What clothes do you wear? How do other people speak and react to you? In what other specific ways does your life change? Picture yourself merging with the perfect you. Know that you already have a gorgeous, slim part inside you who can motivate you to eat healthily, lose weight, and exercise. Press the thumb and index finger of each hand together for fifteen seconds. Take slow, deep breaths, imagining yourself eating healthy food and doing the kind of exercise you love. Picture yourself exercising regularly for one month and enjoying yourself. Relax your fingers and take a few deep breaths.

Press your thumb and index finger together again for fifteen seconds as you make this image strong and vibrant. Become aware of how good you feel. Go forward into the future, focusing on six months from now. See yourself loving your exercise program, being consistent, and looking amazing. Take a few deep breaths. Envisage people you meet telling you how great you look. Sense your confidence increasing. Come back to the present, and relax your index finger and thumb.

Whenever you need motivation during the day, you can press your thumb and index finger together and visualize the perfect you inspiring you to be healthy.

I also have an audio program called *Lose Weight Fast*, which contains several processes that you may like to work with.

Move Your Body

If you have a few extra minutes, stand up, put on some music, and shake your body vigorously for forty seconds. Then slow down and rest for twenty seconds, taking slow, deep breaths. Repeat this exercise five times. This helps activate your metabolism and increases blood circulation. (This is also a great exercise for anyone with circulation problems.)

Perform a Mudra for Weight Loss

This is an amazing mudra, or hand gesture, to help stimulate your metabolism, immune system, and weight loss. (It is also fantastic for any kind of sinus or respiratory condition.)

Clasp your fingers together, except the thumbs. Lift your right thumb toward your head. Touch the tips of your left hand's thumb and index finger, encircling your right thumb. Hold it from two minutes up to twenty minutes to help you lose weight and become healthier. A great time to utilize it is when you are waiting for someone or watching television.

20

HOW YOU CAN HEAL A BROKEN HEART

I have just broken up with my partner, and I feel lost, lonely, sad,
and heavyhearted. Even though the relationship wasn't working, at least I was
somewhat comfortable. Now I'm dealing with the breakup, which makes
me very uncomfortable and tense, and uncertain of how to go on.

Most people go through an experience of rejection or heartbreak at some point in their life. Usually it is a time of confusion, deep emotional pain, and chaos. While it is easy to blame the other person and close your heart, in this chapter, I encourage you to learn from the past, discover a balanced point of view, and find out how love and support is coming into your life in a new form. You have an opportunity to grow and develop from this experience, and become a wiser person, and attract a more suitable relationship into your life.

Breaking Up Is Hard to Do

No matter how difficult a relationship, breaking up often brings up feelings of loss, sadness, grief, loneliness, and uncertainty. It is also common to feel a mixture of anger, fear, rejection, internal conflict, hurt, and disbelief. All of your plans and dreams suddenly begin to disintegrate, and this can be an excruciatingly painful, emotional, and confusing phase.

It can be easy to stay in a relationship that is not working because it is all you know. Feelings of guilt, responsibility, and fear of the future can keep you stuck. When you make a decision to move forward, you will experience discomfort of the unknown. This is where you have an opportunity to review your beliefs and attitudes about yourself, your life, and your relationships. It is a chance to rediscover your own inner strength, heal past wounds, and make new, empowering decisions about the future.

I suggest that you give yourself time for internal exploration, and work with the healing processes at the end of the chapter. If you harbor negative feelings toward your ex-partner, then work with the cord-clearing process from the chapter on creating harmony in your relationships (see page 188).

As this is a very emotional experience, you may also like to experiment with the emotional-release process from the first section (see page 96).

Surrounding Yourself with Support

You need to be particularly gentle with yourself during this time. It is also important to be surrounded by people who love and support you. Many important decisions may have to be made; however, you also need time to express your emotions. It is essential that you do not close up and numb yourself.

It may be helpful to write down your feelings, cry, exercise, be creative, and have some healing treatments that balance your emotions. A relaxing massage, reflexology, acupuncture, aromatherapy, chakra balancing, emotional-release therapy, or other forms of healing treatments can be soothing.

If you don't feel comfortable talking to your friends or family about your breakup, or don't have anyone close around, consider having some counseling sessions. A great counselor can help you acknowledge your feelings and give you a new point of view on your situation.

Supporting Your Children

If you have children, make sure that you talk with them and help them deal with their disappointment, sadness, or hurt. It is vitally important to explain to your children that your decision to separate from their father or mother was not their fault, as children often blame themselves when their parents separate. Make sure you don't talk negatively about your ex, or future ex, with your children. No matter how bad you feel, you do not want to put your child in a position where they have to choose or feel conflicted. If the relationship was extremely abusive and you are concerned about your children's safety, then you must take all the important precautions.

Be aware that your children will have their own relationship with your ex. Having a healthy bond with both parents is extremely important for children's mental, emotional, and physical well-being, as well as their ability to have nourishing relationships with others when they get older.

Learning from the Past

A positive attitude that life will get better can also help you move forward. It is important that you focus on what you can do now rather than on what went wrong in the past. Give yourself permission to take care of yourself and make decisions that help you to move on.

After a breakup, it is imperative that you allow your heart enough time to grieve, and do not close up and lock all the pain inside. You need to heal and learn from past experiences, which can help you move forward and attract a better relationship. If you close up, then you will either stop yourself from meeting someone or keep connecting with a partner who is wrong for you.

Acknowledge the positive aspects of your past relationship, so that you can move forward with a sense of accomplishment and completion rather than failure and disappointment. Spend time reflecting on how you have grown from the experience. What aspects of yourself have you developed? What have you discovered about yourself? How would you like things to be different in your next relationship? What qualities will you be looking for in your next partner?

Take time to discover what you love about yourself, how you want to be treated in a relationship, and how you can have more fun. When you are in pain, it is easy to forget that there are a lot of interesting, loving, creative, soulful people around who can lead you to the most delicious, passionate, profound experience of love. You just need to be open and send out the right vibes.

A Perfect Opportunity to Explore and Transform

If you feel lost, this is a perfect opportunity to begin exploring. Instead of thinking that you know yourself, it is a chance to discover what you like, what attracts you, and what turns you on. You might decide to try things that you have never done, like a dance class, a trip, a job change, or even moving to a new neighborhood or a new city.

After a breakup, one of my clients decided to try pole dancing. She lost weight, gained confidence, and felt sexy. Another client booked a trip to Antarctica and then traveled across South America for three months. She came back refreshed, with a new perspective on life.

I have seen people get out of their box, rediscover their creativity, and make tremendous steps toward their life goals after a separation. It is like they were given a new lease on life. I knew a man who got super fit, ran a marathon, and became an author. Another woman bought a dog, dressed it up, took photos, and made Christmas cards that her friends loved so much that she turned her idea into a multimillion-dollar business. I have heard of people who go back to school, do charity work, become investors, meet their soul mates, and reach a higher level of happiness and fulfillment, all because they had the courage to take a new path and focus on the possibilities, rather than on what they lost.

It is important to understand that what you currently see as an ending is actually a form of transformation. Great questions to ask yourself are *What do I feel I've lost? In what form is life bringing me those qualities now?* For example, if you feel that you have lost affection, who is giving you affection now? It could be a friend or family member, or even someone you met recently who said something kind to you.

If you feel unsupported, look for who is showing you care. It is possible that you are also discovering that you are capable of supporting yourself and becoming more financially empowered. If you feel lonely without your ex, check who is offering to spend time with you. Or maybe you need time out, and this is your opportunity to learn to enjoy your own company. The more you see and acknowledge the new form of what you feel you have lost in your life, the faster you are likely to come back to equilibrium as a full and joyous participant of your life.

Julia's Story: New Beginnings

Julia and Phil lived in Sydney, Australia, for several years and had overcome many challenges to be together. They decided to get married and bought a house where they could start a family. Phil, originally from Greece, decided to visit his family before settling down.

When Phil returned, something wasn't right. He seemed unsettled, confused, and jittery. He told Julia that he wasn't ready to settle down and felt he wanted to go back to Greece to live. Initially, Julia was devastated. Although there had been inklings of Phil's uncertainty about a long-term commitment, Julia did not expect him to be so depressed and unhappy when he returned home. After some internal examination, Julia knew she needed more from the relationship and made the agonizing decision to move out.

Julia moved in with her parents and started looking for another apartment. Her first month on her own was difficult, and she felt lost and alone. However, instead of wallowing in her pain and grief, she decided to focus on what was positive in her life. She reflected on all that she had learned from Phil and realized how much she had grown; she also gained clarity on what she wanted in a new relationship.

Julia spent a few months catching up with friends, rediscovering her old interests, and nurturing herself. She began listening to her intuition and following her heart. Four months after the breakup, Julia was ready to start again. She had a prophetic dream about buying a new apartment, which she purchased a few days later.

Her birthday was coming up, so she got a funky haircut, bought some new clothes, and decided to start dating again. Within a month, Julia met Tom. He was everything that Julia had wanted in a partner: available, caring, attractive, supportive, creative, funny, and completely smitten with her.

I was inspired by Julia's positive attitude and increase in confidence. Once she had processed her pain, she allowed herself to see the new possibilities that life had to offer.

A year and a half later, Julia and Tom got married.

Implicate Order

When I interviewed Dr. John Demartini, author of *The Breakthrough Experience*, he shared, "Whatever we are infatuated with or resentful of consumes space and time in our minds, and we are not free to run our own lives. A balanced perspective allows us to have freedom. The universe has laws that govern equilibrium. When we don't see it, we become disordered. When we see it, we become poised instead of poisoned, present instead of future and past oriented. Wisdom is becoming aware of the implicate order and equilibrium that reigns."[23]

Being on your own gives you an opportunity to find the hidden order and blessings of your experience and recognize that nothing is actually missing; it is just appearing in a different form.

Processes for Healing a Broken Heart

Here are three processes that can help you heal and move forward. Please do the heart-healing process several times. Also, work with the cord-clearing process on page 188 (to clear cords with your ex and anyone else involved) as well as the emotional-release process on page 96 (to release any negative emotions you are experiencing).

Ask Yourself These Powerful Questions

As you work with the following questions, write down the answers so that you can view them later.

What were some of the positive elements that helped me grow in this relationship?

Are there feelings of guilt I am still holding on to that I am willing to release?

Do I need to forgive my ex-partner or myself? (Do the forgiveness exercise from chapter 9 on page 122.)

Who are the people who can offer me support?

Can I give myself permission to receive this support?

Am I willing to keep my heart open, even though it hurts?

What kind of person would I like to attract into my life now?

What kind of relationship would I love to have now?

Recognize the Balance

On one side of a piece of paper, write down what you feel you have lost by breaking up with your partner; on the other side of the paper, write down how those things are appearing in your life now in a new form. Even if they are not obvious, try to recognize the balance in life.

Connect to Your Heart

Place your hands on your chest and take slow, deep breaths. Focus on relaxing your body, and being soft and gentle with yourself.

Say: "Divine Healing Intelligence, please help me to release any anger, sadness, lone-liness, guilt, fear, and _____ add anything else you would like to release) from my heart, mind, body, and energy field. Please help me soothe my heart and fill it with peace, calm, sweetness, softness, and warmth. Bring people into my life who will support and encourage me through this challenging time. Help me with my decision-making processes. Show me the best actions to take to put my life in order. Please bring back feelings of confidence, happiness, and enthusiasm about my future. Thank you."

Repeat the word "CLEAR" several times, until you feel lighter.

Visualize beautiful green, pink, and yellow hues moving through your heart and cleansing it. Now, think about what you would really love to experience, and give yourself permission to receive it.

Complete the process with the following mudra: Sit with a straight back, and bring the palms of your hands together. Hold your hands in a prayer-like position. Bring the tips of your middle fingers to the center of your forehead, at the level of your third-eye chakra. (Your elbows should point out to the sides.) Take slow, deep breaths. Imagine that you are taking back all the power you have given away to your ex. Thank them for the experience of making you stronger. Then hum *ummmmmm* several times. Hold this position for at least two to three minutes, up to five minutes, and do this process two or three times a day after a breakup, until you feel stronger.

21

HOW YOU CAN DEAL WITH GRIEF, DEATH, AND LOSS

*Could you please talk about the different stages of grief when a person
experiences loss? I would also love to hear some inspiration and examples of
handling the death of a loved one, someone really young and someone older.
My grandmother is dying, and I want to do all I can to support her and make
her transition as gentle and loving as possible. Also, my best friend has
recently lost a young child, and I would love to help her deal with that.*

While death and grief are not easy to discuss, every human being has to deal with losing someone they love and, eventually, face their own mortality too. In fact, a great majority would rather have their teeth pulled than discuss it. The possibility of losing a loved one often elicits fear, anxiety, and grief. However, for many people, watching a loved one die can also be life changing. I recently heard a friend share that by witnessing her mother die, she became a free spirit, no longer willing to play by other people's rules. It's like she completely changed her point of view on life and what matters.

Taking the Fear Out of Death

Although it's difficult to watch people we love get ill and die, it is important that we educate ourselves and others about the dying process—to understand that the body is only a shelter for the soul for a relatively brief period. The soul doesn't die; it simply returns to where it came from. In order to make this transition easier, we need to understand the journey of the soul from this reality to the next.

While there are known stages of grief, everyone is unique and experiences the death of a loved one in their own way. While death can feel like a tremendous loss for the people who are left behind, it can also be a beautiful transition and passage into a new reality. In certain cultures, people celebrate death and see it as the soul's return to its true home.

Many people fear death because it is a doorway into the unknown. For people who have experienced past-life regressions or near-death experiences, transitioning into the next phase of their existence is a little less mysterious, and more tranquil.

It is also common for a person to try to communicate with family members and souls who are important to them just before or after his or her death, or even at the moment of death. In my personal life, as well as working with clients, I often witness the process of Soul Communication. Some of the techniques souls can use to reach out to their family involve dreams, movement of objects, flickering lights, touch, visions, mediums, and communications with children.

James Van Praagh, medium and well-known author of books on death and spirit communication, shared, "When you can provide evidence of life after death, and prove to people that there's a survival of consciousness, you take the fear out of death."[24]

My Story: My First Encounter with Death

My first experience with death was completely unexpected. I was pregnant with my first child and enthusiastic about becoming a mother. The pregnancy helped me to connect more with my inner strength.

About three and a half weeks before my baby was due, I saw a midwife at the birth center. She did the usual measurements and told me that everything was perfectly fine. We were about to leave when I had a strong feeling that something was wrong with my baby's heart. The midwife listened to the heartbeat and told me that everything was perfect, and not to worry.

She also told me not to be concerned if the baby wasn't very active, as in the final weeks of pregnancy, there is not much room to move. I accepted her response and went home. A few days later, I noticed that the baby wasn't moving much and I heard strange noises coming from my womb. However, I remembered what the midwife said and waited.

By the end of the week, I started having strong contractions, and Paul drove me to the hospital. The contractions were unbearable, so Paul let me out of the car so that I would get into the hospital quickly. When I walked in, a woman saw me bending over in pain and came over. I leaned on her and she helped me walk. During one of my contractions, she put her hand on my belly and asked when I had last felt the baby move. I could not understand why she asked me this and felt angry.

By the time I got to my hospital room, the contractions had increased, and I felt like the baby was about to come. When the midwife showed up, I was pushing. She helped take the baby out, and I tuned out for a moment, completely exhausted. The room was very quiet. I felt disoriented. I looked up at the midwife and asked, "Is everything all right?"

For a moment, she was quiet, and then said, "I'm sorry." I did not comprehend. I looked at Paul, who had tears in his eyes. My mind went blank. I looked at my baby. He wasn't moving. It hit me.

He was dead.

I asked everyone to leave the room. I could not understand how it happened. This was Australia, after all, and things like this did not happen here as far as I knew. *It was me—something was wrong with me*, I thought. My mind was chaotic. I stared at the ceiling and entered into some kind of a trance. I felt nothing, just frozen.

I don't know how long I stared at the ceiling, but at one point, something incredible happened, and for the first time in my life, I saw an angel. This angel looked kind and beautiful, and she was dressed in white. The angel told me not to worry—that I would have two children soon, a boy and a girl. After she said that, two angelic-looking children appeared next to her. They were beautiful and joyous. I felt a sense of relief and closed my eyes.

For the next few hours, I felt a sense of gratitude. I told Paul that, even though our baby had died, I did not regret the decision to have him, because I had learned so much. I also made a vow that somehow I would use this experience to help others.

This was too big and too painful an experience to disregard. I would honor it and use it for the greater good.

I knew that Paul was devastated and tried to console him. By the morning, my trance began to melt, and pain flooded my body. A hurricane of sorrow and tears engulfed me, and I could no longer reason. All I could do was cry.

The next few weeks were extremely difficult. I felt devastated; not only did I have to deal with my loss and shattered dreams, but also with other people's sympathy and attempts to console Paul and me. Some people shared their stories of loss; others told me horror stories about people losing two, three, even four babies. Hearing this made me feel even more devastated, as there was no way I could handle this again. I did not want to hear any more. All I wanted was to get away and disappear.

My body longed to hold a baby. This feeling, this need, was more painful than anything I had ever experienced.

Paul bought several books on life after death, which we both devoured. However, I still felt distraught. I had nightmares about death and woke up dripping with sweat. Paul decided that we needed help, so we went to see a psychologist. At our first visit, the psychologist told us there was a course we could do that could take us to the edge of death. When I heard this, I knew that I had to do it. Even though it started the same evening and was a five-hour drive away, Paul and I decided to go.

When I walked into the room where the course was being held, I saw about sixty people sitting and talking to each other. I found a chair and sat down. To my surprise, my body started to shudder, and I began to sob. I could not understand my reaction. After all, I had felt completely drained from crying. I had cried so much that I felt like there were no more tears left. Even though I did not know it then, I cried because, on a deep level, I realized that I was not alone—that many other people there were in the same boat, feeling desperate, abandoned, and separated from the Divine.

At the end of that evening, the teacher asked if anyone needed somewhere to stay the night. Paul and I raised our hands. Immediately, a woman offered her place. When I looked into her eyes, I saw the pain and sadness I was feeling. It was like looking into a mirror. I did not know why we needed to stay with her, but I sensed it was important.

When we got to her place, she shared with us that she had lost two children, a baby and a toddler, and her older daughter had recently been raped and was going through a very difficult time. Later, she told us that her husband could not deal with the immense pain and trauma that had afflicted their family, and had left her.

This woman had amazing strength, courage, and softness after having gone through such harrowing experiences. I was speechless and honored to be in her presence; I had no idea where she found the strength to go on.

The following day, we were put into groups of three. I was with a twenty-year-old woman and a twenty-two-year-old man. In the process, we had to imagine that we were three people in a boat, lost at sea but on our way to an island. However, the boat could only carry two people, so to survive, we had to sacrifice a person. To stay in the boat, we had to convince the other two people why we were valuable and deserved to survive. Everyone had to be honest.

The process tested one's self-worth, courage, and will to live. Since, at that point, I wanted to die, I knew I wasn't going to stay in the boat. Once the decision was made, the person who had been rejected had to stare the other people in the eyes without speaking.

For me, this was harder than being thrown overboard because now I had to confront feelings of despair, abandonment, fear, rejection, unworthiness,

259

anger, and shame. I had to face the pain of being separated at birth for a week from my mother, separated from my baby, and feeling separated from Divinity.

Afterward, there was a big forgiveness and letting go process, which was extremely healing.

I knew the next step in my healing journey was to go to a place where I felt at home. I needed to go somewhere special—a place that was holy for me. Paul and I decided to go to Europe. During the trip, we met many people who had lost a child but rarely spoke of it. Hearing their stories allowed me to grieve, and them to acknowledge their loss and start the process of healing. In the United Kingdom, we met Uri Geller, the famous psychic, author, and spoon bender. Uri told us he had experienced the loss of a baby and understood our pain. The meeting was healing and helped us take another step in dealing with our loss.

Paul and I also wrote a lot of poems and songs to express our feelings. And from that, we wrote our first book, *First Kiss*.

Eventually, we had two healthy children.

No one can tell you how to deal with your loss. However, I have found that giving myself permission to feel, talk about, write, and paint helped tremendously. I also discovered that if I could find the blessings in my perceived loss, I could move forward in a more courageous, compassionate, and inspired way.

A few months after we returned from our trip, Paul's mum, who lived in Sydney, invited us to come and stay. The day before we were meant to go, Paul was showering while I was trying to decide what I needed to pack. All of a sudden, I saw an older man standing beside my bed. The man looked familiar, even though I knew I had never met him. Then it dawned on me: it was Paul's maternal grandfather, who had died several years before. After my initial shock subsided, I saw he was holding a baby. He told me not to worry, that he would take good care of our baby. Tears welled up in my eyes; I knew he meant what he said. I was speechless for a moment, and then he disappeared.

260

While visiting Paul's mum, we went to see a medium. The first thing the medium asked us was not to tell him anything. Within moments of tuning in, he started talking about a man who was standing behind Paul. He described the man I had seen several days earlier. I asked if the man was holding anything. At first, the medium said he held one red rose. (Paul's grandmother's name was Rose.) A moment later, we watched as his eyes welled up with tears. I knew he had seen our baby. Softly, he said, "He is holding a baby." Paul's grandfather shared an almost identical message with the psychic as he had shared with me.

This experience not only confirmed what I had seen but also helped me deal with my grief.

Stages of Grief

As I mentioned earlier, there are several well-recognized stages of grief. It is important to understand that these occur at different times, and each is unique for a bereaved person. The order can also vary vastly. A huge part of moving through grief can depend on an individual's beliefs and education, so some people may skip stages while others linger in a particular phase.

Shock and Denial

Often, the first stage is shock and denial. Shock can offer protection from being overwhelmed and going into a complete meltdown. Denial can be seen as one's refusal to accept reality. It is important to be aware of this stage and know that it will eventually pass, without getting stuck in it.

Pain and Guilt

When the shock wears off, it can be replaced by severe emotional, mental, and physical pain. Allow yourself to experience the waves of pain, and cry, scream, breathe deeply, punch a pillow, sing, shake, or box in order to release the charge. The most damaging thing is to suppress the pain, or to try to escape it through drugs, alcohol, or violence.

261

You may also experience feelings of guilt or remorse, believing that you did not do enough or could have done something differently. You need to be gentle and forgive yourself for whatever you think you did wrong.

Anger

Anger can manifest against Divinity, yourself, fate, medicine, doctors, family members, and other perceived perpetrators, especially in the case of murder. The most common questions are *Why me? What is wrong with me? What have I done wrong? Why am I being punished?* It is very important that you express this anger in healthy ways, through emotional-release processes, writing, painting, boxing, dancing, singing, playing sports, or working with an appropriate health professional or body worker.

Bargaining

Bargaining typically involves trying to make a deal with whatever Higher Intelligence a person believes in. It can include making vows never to drink, smoke, abuse, lie, or gamble. It can also entail making promises to Divinity to get clean, help others, be of service, return to study, look after your health, dedicate your life to Divinity, and so forth.

Although bargaining does not bring someone back to life, occasionally, when a person is gravely ill or in a life-or-death situation, asking for Divine help can create miracles. I have also observed people changing their lives after making particularly strong vows or promises to transform.

Sadness, Depression, and Loneliness

Sadness, depression, and loneliness are normal stages of grief that can occur at different times in your life, even years after a loved one has passed. These feelings may last for minutes, or linger for weeks or months. You may feel empty, alone, and lost.

Rather than suppressing those feelings, you may listen to a song that helps you remember your loved one; write down your memories; meditate on what was special about this person; or see a grief counselor, or even a well-regarded medium or healer, who can give you closure.

It can be useful to reflect on the qualities you feel you have lost because this person is no longer with you. Also, try to see who in your life now displays the same or similar traits and qualities.

Understanding that the life of a soul continues after death, and that you will reconnect with your family and friends when you pass over, can help tremendously in dealing with feelings of loss.

Moving Forward

During the moving-forward stage, you begin to focus on making the best of your life and looking for ways to heal. You may do some self-help or healing seminars, read spiritual books, contemplate your life choices, and change your values.

You may decide to travel, move, change jobs, return to school, or reconsider your relationships. You then have a possibility to re-enter life with a more positive, uplifting perspective—to embrace new experiences and live each day to the fullest.

It is important to not make any rash decisions but to instead move forward step by step.

Acceptance and Peace

For a person who is dying, acceptance may come when he or she makes peace with earthly life and decides to move on. Usually it's a process of reflection and forgiveness in which they acknowledge their contribution in life and express their love to family and friends.

For the people who are left behind, acceptance can occur at any moment, once they realize their loved one is now free of pain and suffering, and that he or she has entered a better place.

Sarah's Story: A Friend's Transition

Sarah called me because her friend Delta was dying of cancer, and she wanted to know if I could help Delta's transition.

I agreed to tune in. When I focused on Delta, I saw an image of a female lying motionless in bed. Sarah confirmed that Delta was in a coma. I saw a young boy next to her, who I immediately felt was her son. I could tell that Delta's soul was held in her body by a thread. Telepathically, Delta relayed that she was concerned about how her death would affect her son, and was holding on until she felt he could accept it and forgive her for leaving him. She wanted me to relay to him that she would always be around, watching over and helping him from the spirit world. Sarah was grateful for the information and thanked me profusely.

I hung up the phone and went downstairs. All of a sudden, an image of the Star of David appeared in front of my eyes. The image was persistent, and I felt that it related to Delta, so I called Sarah, who informed me that Delta was Jewish. I had a sense that, for Delta, the Star of David was an important symbol. Sarah promised to take her own Star of David and place it on Delta's chest.

A few hours later, Sarah called to tell me that when she went to see Delta, she found that she already wore a Star of David pendant. Nevertheless, Sarah placed her pendant on her friend's heart. Within moments, she noticed a tear streaming down Delta's face. It was like Delta acknowledged that she had been heard.

Soon after, Delta's son came into the room and told his mother that it was okay for her to move on. Within moments, her heart stopped.

A few weeks later, Sarah came to me for a healing session. Within minutes, Delta appeared in the room, but I decided not to mention it to Sarah. I saw that Delta came to her, hugged her, and proceeded to hold Sarah's feet. I asked Sarah if she felt anything, and she told me that she felt like her feet were on fire. I shared with Sarah that Delta was right beside her, which was a huge comfort. Then Delta communicated some important personal and accurate details about Sarah to me. Sarah was extremely grateful for the infromation. It was a very touching experience.

My Grandmother's Story: Transition

Though I have already shared examples of dying and dealing with grief, I cannot complete this chapter without writing about my grandmother's passing. Her transition was an incredibly difficult and healing experience, and I feel that many readers would find it quite illuminating.

Two months before she died, my grandmother was diagnosed with leukemia. Since my grandmother had survived World War II, where she lost her mother and seven siblings, I was not surprised that her blood was deeply affected. In fact, I had already met many people who had been afflicted with this disease after surviving the war. In a way, I was almost surprised that my grandmother didn't get cancer until she was in her eighties.

Since she was a fighter, most people in my family were in shock when they heard the news of her illness. There was a lot of talk about her beating this, getting better, and living longer. It was really hard to accept that she was dying, as she looked so strong and energetic, and had an insatiable thirst for life.

After my initial anger with the doctor for telling us that she had only a few months to live, I decided to take his prediction as a gift. I saw it as an opportunity to spend quality time with my grandmother, and I felt that I had a chance to help her and others in the family heal.

I encouraged my grandmother to focus on her own healing and appreciation of life. My intention was to help her transcend the suffering she had experienced and find peace.

In her last month of life, my grandmother was the most positive, open, and receptive that I had ever known her to be. She had let go of her resistance, anxiety, and concerns, and listened to me with an open heart and mind. I taught her exercises for pain relief, emotional release, changing negative thinking, and healing the past. She was also open to talking about angels and was willing to connect with her deceased parents.

I saw her almost daily in those last months, and we shared many special moments. When I asked if there was anything she regretted or wished she had done differently, she looked at me in an intense way and decidedly said, "No."

Two nights before my grandmother died, I tuned in and saw that her soul was halfway out of her body.

That night, we were still able to speak with her and make her laugh. What fascinated me was that, when she spoke, I saw her mother's spirit standing behind her on her left and her father's spirit on her right. I knew that they were there to support her on her journey to the other side. This made me feel comforted.

The following day, my grandmother was taken to the hospital, as she had developed pneumonia. Within a few hours, she was unconscious. When my cousin, mother, husband, and I were driving to the hospital, I saw my grandmother's soul. She shared how much she loved and appreciated each of us and asked us to look after my grandfather.

When we got to the hospital, I talked to my grandmother about letting go as she moved in and out of consciousness. She could no longer talk to me, but I knew she was listening. At one point, I saw her parents with several of her siblings standing near her bed.

Her soul seemed calm, and she told me that she felt lighter. However, her body was still fighting. During the night, my cousin Jenny asked how my grandmother's soul managed to go in and out of her body. Just then, I saw a cord that was still connecting her soul to her body. This fascinated me, as I hadn't realized that her soul could not disconnect from her body until the body died and the cord was dissolved. It seemed fitting: when we come into this life, we have a cord attached to our mother that has to be cut, and when we leave our bodies, we have a cord that is attached to our bodies that we have to let go of.

I saw my grandmother's soul get confused when she realized she could not come back into her dying body and she could not go to the spirit world, as the cord still connected her to her body. I explained that it was okay—that she was moving on—but it was going to take a bit of time.

The next morning, her breathing became more and more labored. I could no longer stay in the room and asked Jenny to come downstairs with me. We were waiting for my brother when I saw my grandmother's soul. I asked her if she was waiting for my grandfather. She nodded but seemed a bit unsure. I told her that we would look after him and that it was time for her to go. She was silent for a moment, then turned to me and said, "OK, Inochka (a sweet way of saying my name in Russian). I'll go then."

I knew then that it was time to go upstairs to her room. We raced there and saw a nurse standing next to her bed. She told us that we were just in time to see our grandmother take her last breaths. We watched, sending her enormous love and telling her we loved her, over and over. It was a sad but liberating experience.

Taking a Divine Perspective

After my grandmother died, I heard someone say, "There is no loss in reality." This was another way of relating to death—as a return home. From the Divine perspective, there is never any loss; there is just a movement, a takeoff from one dimension to another.

I also realized that although my grandmother was physically absent, if I was open and receptive, I would find many of her loving qualities in other people.

Since her death, I have met several people who have given me deep love and support. Although they do not replace my grandmother, each time someone is loving, caring, and courageous, I am reminded of my grandmother and feel deeply grateful.

When a person you are close to is dying, it can give you an opportunity to open your heart and unlock your emotions in a way that you have never allowed. It is a chance to go deeper and express your appreciation for the person who is transitioning, feel the fullness of your love and grow spiritually. It is a time to slow down, reflect, go within, and explore.

When we are confronted with death, there are many questions that come up about our own mortality and how we live our lives. It is a chance to discover what really matters to us.

A Gift to the Dying

When someone close to you is dying, the biggest gift you can give is your time, love, and compassion. This person needs to feel significant and have the chance to acknowledge his or her life and contribution. Go and see your loved one, and talk. If they are in a coma, have Alzheimer's, or another condition that prevents speaking, communicate with them anyway. They can still hear you, even if they cannot answer.

Educating people about the soul and the spirit world can also significantly lessen their fear of dying.

Processes for Handling Death

The following three processes can help you to support someone who is dying, and address your own fear and loss. I recommend that you work with the emotional-release process on page 96 as well. My previous book, *The Secret Language of Your Body*, also has a lot of processes that can help you to deal with various emotions, and even help you to forgive a person who has died.

Pray

When you are near a loved one who is dying, take the time to say a loving prayer. If you can, place your hands on the person's heart with the intention of sending him or her love, care, and support. Say something like, "Angels, Guides, and Divine helpers please surround _____ (say the name of the person), with love, care, and light. Please assist _____ (say the name of the person) to transition in the softest, easiest, most comfortable way possible. Take them to the light with ease and grace at the appropriate moment. Thank you."

The intention here is to make the dying person feel comfortable and at peace. If several family members are gathered when someone is dying or in a coma, then share your most memorable moments about the person who is transitioning. If you need to forgive them or be forgiven, then this is the best time to do so.

Work with the section on emotional healing in this book to release all the grief and painful feelings that come up.

Shock Release

If you are in a state of deep fear, shock, or trauma, do the following process. This mudra helps the nervous system to relax and the immune system to stabilize.

Encircle your left ring finger with the four fingers of your right hand. Extend the right thumb into the middle of your left hand, applying a substantial amount of pressure.

Say: "I now give myself permission to release all fear and shock from my body and cellular memories, and to unwind, calm down, and relax. I am loved and supported. From this moment, things are improving, getting better and lighter."

Repeat the word "CLEAR" several times, until you feel lighter.

Hold this position for five to ten minutes, then swap hands. Focus on breathing deeply and relaxing. Visualize green light moving through your nervous system and releasing any shock.

Work with Fear

The death of a loved one can bring up a lot of fear and uncertainty. This is a simple exercise that can be helpful to let go of fear:

Write down what you are afraid of. Number your fears, from the worst thing that could happen to the smaller fears. Do this slowly. Then give yourself a moment; sit and feel each fear intensely. What is it that you don't want to experience?

Place your hands on the part of your body where you feel the most fear. Take some slow, deep breaths. Become aware of any uncomfortable sensations.

Say to yourself or aloud: "I am willing to let this fear go."

Imagine being able to take this sensation of fear out of your body and into the palms of your hands. Imagine that the fear becomes a bird. Surrender the bird to a higher source and visualize it flying away.

Say a Healing Statement

Say: "Divine Wisdom, please give me the understanding of how this really challenging situation can also help me grow, evolve, and move forward in life. Please give me the loving guidance I require to surrender my fear of loss, and the guidance to allow me to recognize the balance of life and Divine support I have in the face of death. Help me come to terms with my loss and see it as a transformation. Bring me the people who will understand me, have compassion, and help me heal. Please show me the blessings of this experience and give me hope. Thank you."

Repeat the word "SURRENDER" several times, until you feel lighter.

I ask you to use the word *surrender* instead of *clear* because, when the situation is challenging and beyond our understanding, the only thing we can do is surrender it to a higher source.

CONCLUSION

I hope that *The Secret of Life Wellness* has expanded your awareness with regard to some of life's most interesting and challenging subjects. Throughout these pages I have shared many stories from my own experiences, as well as those of clients, family, and friends. I hope that these accounts have given you a lot of insights into your life, and have motivated you to make new and empowering choices.

While reading a book can inspire you, nothing beats practicing the processes described. If you turn to page 277, you will find a section titled "An Ongoing Practice." I encourage you to read it and follow the suggestions, or create your own daily practice. Your life will only improve if you take positive action. Although many of the subjects I have explored are quite serious, laughter and joy are vital parts of life. Thus, when you are creating your wellness plan, make sure that it has plenty of variety, creativity, and fun!

If you have found this book useful, I encourage you to share it with the people you know. Even if your family or friends have different points of view, it can make for a

271

lively and interesting discussion. You might even be surprised to find out how open to healing and spirituality they are.

As I hope is evident from this book, some of my greatest joy comes from teaching Visionary Intuitive Healing® workshops around the world. If you are drawn to experience a live or an online seminar, I encourage you to check my website, InnaSegal.com. I'm constantly exploring new ways of giving people access to powerful and transformational tools, so feel free to connect with me through my website, blog, or social media.

I would love to find out how *The Secret of Life Wellness* has changed your life. Please feel free to email your experiences to Inna@InnaSegal.com

I wish you an incredible and inspiring life journey!

love
Inna

ACKNOWLEDGMENTS

First and foremost, I am deeply grateful to my husband, Paul, who is the most loving, kind, and supportive person I know. I could not do all that I do if he were not there to guide me, support me, and inspire me. No matter what challenge I am dealing with, he is willing to listen, give me a new perspective, and help me move forward. His wisdom and patience are truly incredible. Paul, I love you from the depth of my heart and soul. You are my angel.

I am blessed to have two incredibly wise and loving children. Raphael, I adore you; you make me so proud. I love your sensitivity; your care; and your ability to listen, be open, and ask deep questions. You are growing up to be a remarkable person. Angelina, you bring light everywhere you go. You are the queen of compliments. You are bigger than life, incredibly smart, loving, funny, and extraordinary, a true gift.

I am profoundly thankful to my parents. I always feel loved, accepted, and supported by you. Thank you for everything you have done and do for my family.

ACKNOWLEDGMENTS

I am grateful to all the wonderful people who are part of my family. I especially want to acknowledge my brother, Marat, who has inspired me to look after my physical body better and to train regularly. I love you!

To my cousin Jenny, I am so grateful to share my journey with you. Thank you for your patience, willingness to listen, and your enthusiasm for my work. You know you are very special. Also, to my cousin Yuri; his wife, Mandy; and their daughter, Emily; I love observing how your family is growing.

I would like to acknowledge my grandparents Emma and Misha, who are now looking out for my family from the spirit world. How you have lived your life, your courage, your love, and your simplicity is my greatest inspiration.

To some of my close friends, Piotr Miklaszewski, Adam Jones, Frédéric Edinval, Carlos Muñoz, Juan Manuel Guiterrez, Marina and Paul Loza, Myriam Quiñones Pescador, Sandrine Marechal, Katia Loisel-Furey, and LeGrande Green, thank you for all you do to make my life joyful, meaningful, and fun. Your constant care and willingness to go out of your way are very touching. My heartfelt thanks also goes to the people who have supported me since my work has come out in the United States: Reverend Michael Beckwith, thank you for your inspirational foreword, interviewing me on your radio show, and the love and support you have given me. Reverend Nirvana Reginald Gayle, thank you for believing in me, taking time to share your wisdom and being my friend. Reverend Kevin Ross, your enthusiasm about my work from the first time we spoke was extremely uplifting. Scott Wilson from HeartThreads clothing, it's been a joy to get to know you and work with you. Simran Singh of 11:11 Talk Radio, thank you for your faith in me and for sharing my work.

I am also incredibly grateful to all the people who have organized my workshops all over the world—in particular, Sandrine Marechal in France: your faith in my work is very moving, and I am so thankful for the work that you do to help people heal. I also want to acknowledge Myriam Quiñones Pescador, who has traveled all around Mexico, France, and Spain with me, and has encouraged countless people to use my healing work, has done thousands of healing sessions, has taught many workshops based on *The Secret Language of Your Body* and Visionary Intuitive Healing®, and has translated my work into Spanish. You are an amazing friend, healer, and teacher; I don't know if I can find the words to thank you. I am also extremely grateful to Nuria Borrayo and Kriss Sepúlveda de Jolly and many others for all their incredible help and support in Mexico.

Another special acknowledgement goes to Dianne Wynne: you are a pleasure to work with. I am constantly inspired and humbled by your enthusiasm, persistence, and vibrancy.

I also feel a lot of appreciation for all my organizers from around the world.

Thank you to my musical director, Phillip Gelbach, for your heartfelt and talented contribution to the Visionary Intuitive Healing® audio programs and audio downloads accompanying this book.

I want to express my deepest gratitude to my clients and workshop participants. You have given me the amazing gift of opening my heart and contributing to your lives.

I am extremely grateful to have been guided and supported by Cynthia Black, co-founder of Beyond Words Publishing, who will always be an inspiration to me.

Thank you to Richard Cohn for your generosity and advice. I love having Beyond Words as my publisher. Thanks to Judith Curr at Atria Books for your encouragement and support. To the rest of the team at Beyond Words—Tim Schroeder, Emily Han, Sheila Ashdown, Lindsay S. Brown, Emmalisa Sparrow, Henry Covey, Devon Smith, Bill Brunson, Whitney Quon, Ruth Hook, Jessica Sturges, and Leah Brown—thank you for your commitment to making this the best book possible.

I am also incredibly thankful to Lisa Keim at Simon & Schuster and Sylvia Hayse at Beyond Words for the incredible work you do enabling my books to be translated into many languages around the world.

I can't say enough positive things about working with the Beyond Words team. I am so touched by how generous, accommodating, and thoughtful you are.

Lastly, I would like to offer my deepest gratitude to all the publishers, editors, designers and publicists around the world who make this book available to so many people who are seeking to improve their well-being.

APPENDIX

An Ongoing Practice

This book—and all my work—has been created to encourage you to lead a healing life-style. This means that every day of your life is dedicated to being loving to yourself and others. Even if you lead a busy lifestyle, you can find a few minutes throughout your day to connect to yourself and improve your life.

I believe that a daily practice that enhances your well-being is extremely important. Although you can create your own practice, I want to give you a few suggestions that you can do each day based on what you are working on in your life:

Start each day with the protection/purification process in chapter 8, "How You Can Connect to Divine Energy and Protect Yourself." Page 114.

Do the space-clearing exercise anytime you feel heavy or strange energy in your house or workplace. If you see a lot of people, do it daily. Otherwise, once or twice a week is sufficient. Page 217.

If, in the morning or during the day, you feel any unpleasant emotions, do the emotional-release process from chapter 6, page 96. I have refined and deepened this process so it is extremely powerful. It is really important that you release negative emotions as fast as possible, before they do any damage. If you are working with *The Secret Language of Your Body*, you can also integrate specific emotions and colors during this process.

If you have had a recent shock or trauma, do the "Shock Release," "Work with Fear," and "Say a Healing Statement" processes from chapter 21, "How You Can Deal with Grief, Death, and Loss." Pages 268–270.

If you experience anxiety, or feel ready to forgive your family and heal the past, work with your inner child. The inner-child process in chapter 3 is extremely important, and I suggest you start with it (page 47). Also, you can purchase and work regularly with my audio program called *Healing Your Inner Child*.

If you need to forgive someone, do the "Practice Forgiveness" exercise in the "Process for Loving Unconditionally" section in chapter 9. Page 122.

If you are working on opening your heart, do all the processes from chapter 2 (pages 32–33), "How You Can Love Yourself" (page 21), and work on your heart chakra from chapter 5, "How You Can Use Your Energy Centers to Heal and Spiritually Evolve," on page 71.

If your aim is to lose weight, practice the processes described in chapter 19 for five to seven days a week, until you feel happy with your weight. Pages 242–245.

Work with the chakras regularly—it only takes a few minutes to work with each one. Connect to at least three each week. Pages 64–83.

If you are ready to live your soul's purpose, do the exercises for soul connection from chapter 7 (page 108), as well as those for discovering your soul's purpose in chapter 12 (page 164). Do these at least three to four times a week, until you have more clarity.

If you want to focus on creating success and abundance, do the exercises from chapter 18, "How You Can Create More Money and Success in Your Life." Do these daily for at least three months. If you can't do all of them, just practice what you can. Pages 228–232.

Exercises such as past-life regression (page 150), increasing your intuition (page 16), connecting to soul mates (page 139), attracting a relationship (page 177), healing a broken heart (page 252), preparing for pregnancy (page 198), and handling death (page 268) can be done whenever you are going through a related experience and are drawn to work on these.

Even if you are not in a relationship, or if you feel that yours is fantastic, please read about and practice the "Perform a Cord Clearing" exercise from chapter 14. It is one of the most powerful exercises to improve issues in all types of relationships. Page 188.

Although you may not be pregnant, I encourage you to read the chapter on pregnancy and birth—chapter 15—in order to understand more about your own birth. Page 191.

If you have children, do the healing processes in chapter 16 nightly or several times a week as a family. Also, encourage your children to participate and use their own imaginations. Page 210.

I wish you all the best with your journey of wellness and look forward to hearing about your progress.

NOTES

1. Mona Lisa Schulz, *Awakening Intuition* (New York: Three Rivers Press, 1998), 31.

2. Deepak Chopra, *Reinventing the Body, Resurrecting the Soul* (London: Rider, 2009), 39.

3. Steven Thayer, quoted by Leon Pelletier and Phoenix Rising Star in "Cellular Memory—Cell Level Healing," *The Spirit of Ma'at*, September 2007: http://spiritofmaat.com/sep07/cellular_memory.html.

4. Deepak Chopra, *Reinventing the Body, Resurrecting the Soul* (London: Rider, 2009), 37.

5. See A. Siegman et al., *Journal of Behavioral Medicine* 21, no. 4 (1998). See also D. Carroll et al., *Journal of Epidemiology and Community Health* (September 1998).

6. Ronald Grossarth-Maticek and Hans J. Eysenck, *Behaviour Research and Therapy* 29, no. 1 (1991).

7. Glen Rein, Mike Atkinson, and Rollin McCraty, *Journal of Advancement in Medicine* 8, no. 2 (1995): 87–105.

8. Candace B. Pert, Ph.D., *Molecules of Emotion* (New York: Scribner, 1997), 18–19.

9. Deepak Chopra, *Quantum Healing* (New York: Bantam, 1989), 41.

10. Patrick Quanten, "Healing versus Curing," *Active Health*, August 2002: http://freespace.virgin.net/ahcare.qua/literature/mindspirit/healingvscuring.html (accessed April 17, 2013).

11. Robin Youngson, quoted by Inna Segal in *The Secret Language of Your Body* (Hillsboro, OR: Beyond Words/Atria Books, 2010), ii.

12. Petrea King (founding director of the Quest for Life Centre), in discussion with the author, February 2009.

13. Helen Schucman and William T. Thetford, *A Course in Miracles* (Course in Miracles Society, 1972), 3.

14. Caroline Myss, quoted by Inna Segal in "Healthy Choices for a Healing Lifestyle," *Living Now*, July 2002.

15. Richard Bach (author of *Jonathan Livingston Seagull*), in discussion with the author, June 2002.

16. Paolo Coelho (author of *The Alchemist)*, in discussion with the author, October 2002.

17. Ibid.

18. Masaru Emoto, *The Miracle of Water* (New York: Simon & Schuster, 2007).

19. Suze Orman (author of *The 9 Steps to Financial Freedom*), in discussion with the author, May 2004.

20. Robert Kiyosaki (author of *Rich Dad, Poor Dad*), in discussion with the author, May 2002.

21. Ibid.

22. Todd Tucker, *The Great Starvation Experiment* (Minneapolis: University of Minnesota Press, 2008).

23. John Demartini (author of *The Breakthrough Experience*), in discussion with the author, September 2004.

24. James Van Praagh (author of *Growing Up in Heaven*), in discussion with the author, June 2004.

ABOUT THE AUTHOR

Inna Segal is the creator of Visionary Intuitive Healing® and the bestselling, award-winning author of *The Secret Language of Your Body: The Essential Guide to Health and Wellness* and *The Secret Language of Color Cards*. She is also an internationally recognized healer, professional speaker, author, and television host. Inna's clients include doctors, CEOs, healthcare professionals, actors, and sports personalities.

Inna is a gifted healer and a pioneer in the field of energy medicine and human consciousness. She can "see" illness and blocks in a person's body by intuitive means, explain what is occurring, and guide people through self-healing processes.

When Inna was a teenager, she suffered from severe back pain that continued to deteriorate, despite visits to doctors, chiropractors, and other healthcare professionals. By her early twenties, Inna's pain was so intense that she was barely able to walk.

In an incredible twist of fate, Inna, while meditating, discovered an unusual way of communicating with her body. By tuning in to her back and releasing all the pain and negative emotions, she was able to heal herself.

Inna now dedicates herself to assisting others in their journey of self-healing and empowerment. Her practical healing techniques, healing frequency, internet presence, and radio and television appearances are changing the lives of millions of people all around the world.

Inna travels worldwide to teach Visionary Intuitive Healing® programs, she is available as a keynote speaker or a presenter at conferences, events, book clubs, and bookstore events. You can contact Inna via email at Inna@InnaSegal.com.

For further insight on Inna, please visit www.InnaSegal.com

Resources Available from the Author

The Secret Language of Your Body: The Essential Guide to Health & Wellness
The Secret Language of Color Cards

Visionary Intuitive Healing® Audio Programs

Create Perfect Health
Success, Money & Prosperity
Affirmations for Happiness, Confidence & Well-Being
Lose Weight Fast
Nine Chakras: The Secret to Health, Clarity & Freedom
Healing Your Inner Child
The Secret Language of Your Emotions: Volumes 1 & 2
Peaceful Sleep
Accelerated Learning & Memory Enhancement
Freedom from Pain
Freedom from Stress
Experience Youthful Clear Skin
Healing Meditation for Children (Raphael Alexander Segal)
Colour Healing Meditations for Children (Raphael & Angelina Segal)
Become a Money Magnet: 30-Day Program
Right Now (inspirational songs)

Visionary Intuitive Healing® Transformative Music

Gateway: A Musical Journey into the Light
Tantric Music for Heart & Soul
Spa Sensations Music
Reflexology & Relaxation Music
Tranquillity: Rest, Relax & Rejuvenate

Peaceful Sleep Music
Accelerated Learning & Memory Enhancement Music
Animal Healing & Relaxation

For further information and free audio samples, please visit: www.InnaSegal.com

Visionary Intuitive Healing® Transformative Courses

The Secret of Life Wellness (2-day course)

"The Secret of Life Wellness" is designed to help you develop your intuition, reclaim your inner power, love yourself, and deal with challenging emotions. Discover your value, and give yourself the love and nourishment you deserve. Connect and communicate with your soul. Learn to recognize and attract soul mates. Discover and start to live your soul purpose. Improve your relationships with others. Stop sabotaging your progress and create success in your life. Create your best life with a combination of simple, easy, fast, effective, and deeply transformational processes.

The Secret Language of Your Body (2-day course)

"The Secret Language of Your Body" is an essential workshop for you to discover how to energize your body, release pain, undo negative patterns in minutes, and become vibrantly well. You will be guided to strengthen your immune system, revitalize your nervous system, and clear stress and tension from your body. This course is for you if you have read *The Secret Language of Your Body*, found it effective, and are ready to completely transform your health by receiving the messages your body desires to give you. You will be amazed at how some simple techniques can create more ease, freedom, and joy in your life.

The Secret Language of Your Emotions (2-day course)

In this workshop, you have an opportunity to not only understand how your emotions affect your health and your ability to live a happy, deep empowered life, but how you can also work to release limiting, heavy, traumatic feelings. Discover how to experience more ease, flow, opportunity, flexibility, depth of feeling, and clarity in your life. Purify and give birth to a new, more peaceful, happy, and balanced you.

The Secrets of Your Shadow Revealed (2–3-day course)

This exciting and unique workshop will change your life and help you to embrace the gifts of your shadow side. You will discover how to free yourself from stagnation, victimhood, guilt, and self-sabotage. In a world where we are striving for perfection yet are constantly bombarded by fear campaigns, this workshop will demonstrate how you can turn your limitations into strengths. Discover how all the parts of yourself that you don't like and reject actually contain enormous gifts. You can transform a life of struggle, worry, and pain into a life of freedom, inner peace, confidence, and ease.

Visionary Intuitive Healing*—Level 1 (5- to 6-day course)

If you are ready to connect to the Divine and discover real freedom, you will love this life-changing workshop. This is like nothing else you have ever experienced. You will learn how to heal mental, emotional, and energetic blockages, and pain in people and animals. Intensify your intuitive abilities. Work with your nine main chakras. Tune in to another person's energy and receive messages. Let go of toxic blocks and emotions. Clear negative core beliefs. Transform your personal relationships. Clear outdated agreements and vows. Discover the laws of the universe, and how to work with these to become prosperous in every area of your life.

Further Visionary Intuitive Healing* transformative courses

Success, Money & Prosperity (*2–3-day course*)
The Secret Language of Your Intuition (*2-day course*)
The Secrets of Your Destiny Revealed (*4-day course*)
Quantum Leap: Sharpening Your Skills (*3–4-day course*)
Visionary Intuitive Healing—Level 2 (*5- to 6-day course*)
Visionary Intuitive Healing—Level 3 (*5- to 6-day course*)

If you would like information on attending Visionary Intuitive Healing® training programs or to book Inna Segal for a presentation, please visit www.InnaSegal.com.